SBAs and EMQs for
Human Disease (Medicine)
in Dentistry

T0177739

SBAs and EMQs for Human Disease (Medicine) in Dentistry

Oluyori K. Adegun BDS MSc CILT MFDS RCS(Ed) PhD PGCAP FHEA

Honorary Clinical Senior Lecturer in Clinical Human Health and Disease, Institute of Dentistry, Bart's and London School of Medicine and Dentistry, Queen Mary, University of London
Speciality Registrar in Oral and Maxillofacial Pathology, University College London Hospitals NHS Foundation Trust

John A.G. Buchanan Hons BSc MSc MB BS FDS RCPS (OM) Glasg FDS RCS Eng. FRCP

Clinical Senior Lecturer/Honorary Consultant in Oral Medicine and Lead for Quality Assurance at Bart's and The London School of Medicine and Dentistry, Queen Mary University of London/Bart's Health NHS Trust

Farida Fortune MB BS FDS RCS Eng. FRCP PhD CBE

Professor of Medicine in Relation to Oral Health/Honorary Consultant in Oral Medicine, Clinical and Diagnostic Oral Sciences, Bart's and The London School of Medicine and Dentistry, Queen Mary, University of London

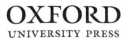

OXFORD
UNIVERSITY PRESS

OXFORD
UNIVERSITY PRESS

Great Clarendon Street, Oxford, OX2 6DP,
United Kingdom

Oxford University Press is a department of the University of Oxford.
It furthers the University's objective of excellence in research, scholarship,
and education by publishing worldwide. Oxford is a registered trade mark of
Oxford University Press in the UK and in certain other countries

First Edition published in 2021

Impression: 1

Published in the United States of America by Oxford University Press
198 Madison Avenue, New York, NY 10016, United States of America

British Library Cataloguing in Publication Data
Data available

Library of Congress Control Number: 2020950283

ISBN 978-0-19-880099-6

Printed and bound by
CPI Group (UK) Ltd, Croydon, CR0 4YY

Oxford University Press makes no representation, express or implied, that the
drug dosages in this book are correct. Readers must therefore always check
the product information and clinical procedures with the most up-to-date
published product information and data sheets provided by the manufacturers
and the most recent codes of conduct and safety regulations. The authors and
the publishers do not accept responsibility or legal liability for any errors in the
text or for the misuse or misapplication of material in this work. Except where
otherwise stated, drug dosages and recommendations are for the non-pregnant
adult who is not breast-feeding

Links to third party websites are provided by Oxford in good faith and
for information only. Oxford disclaims any responsibility for the materials
contained in any third party website referenced in this work.

PREFACE

Throughout the world, advances in medicine combined with an ageing population and an increasing emphasis on healthcare delivery as an outpatient and in primary care has resulted in an increasing number of patients with complex medical conditions—who are also taking multiple medications—seeking dental treatment from dental care practitioners in general practice. Whereas previously these patients would have been treated on an inpatient basis, there is an increasing emphasis on outpatient treatment.

These changing trends underline the importance that dental healthcare providers in both general and specialty practice have a sound and up-to-date knowledge of human disease (medicine) in dentistry and clinical pharmacology and therapeutics.

During the years of teaching human disease (medicine) in dentistry to undergraduate dental students, we have regularly been asked to recommend reading and self-assessment resources for self-directed learning to facilitate preparation for examinations. For the former a repertoire of textbooks, case reports, and serial journal articles specifically written for medicine in dentistry exists. However, for the latter there remains no specifically prepared self-assessment material to refer students to. This impacts on their ability to engage in formative learning, reflect, and identify their learning needs, as well as prepare for their all-important summative examinations. To address this gap, we have written a dedicated self-assessment material, which:

- Is presented using current assessment formats (i.e. SBAs and EMQs), which are currently considered to be the formats of choice for integrated knowledge tests on the human disease (medicine) in dentistry
- Covers specific learning outcomes for the human disease course as outlined in the General Dental Council's (GDC) Preparing for Practice document
- Incorporates clinical scenarios designed to test the recognition of oral and systemic signs and symptoms, and selection of the most appropriate investigations and management, all of which should foster the development of clinical problem-solving skills
- Facilitates formative learning by ensuring each question is accompanied by the answer and the rationale using clear facts explaining why the correct response is right and why the other responses are less plausible. This approach will help evaluate individual learning needs thereby identifying areas which may require further reading
- Is written by specialists experienced in the design and delivery of the human disease (medicine) in dentistry curriculum and are familiar with the common presentations, pathologies, and dilemmas encountered while working within the specialty

We hope that you will find this formative assessment resource to be stimulating and interesting and that it will help you to develop the necessary knowledge base, problem-solving, and clinical skills required to deliver high-quality and safe patient care in your everyday practice as a dental healthcare practitioner. It also anticipated that exposure to a variety of clinical signs and symptoms from the different systems in the body while using this book will contribute towards the knowledge of the most appropriate clinical specialty to refer a patient to for further care.

Oluyori K. Adegun, John A.G. Buchanan, and Farida Fortune

ACKNOWLEDGEMENTS

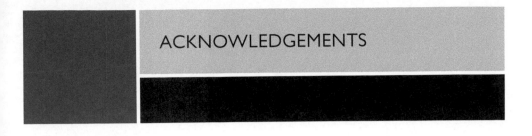

We would like to thank the editorial staff of Oxford University Press who encouraged us to produce this self-test learning resource in which we have endeavoured to incorporate clinical scenarios designed to test reasoning skills and develop the cognitive processes required to navigate the complexities of medicine in relation to dentistry. We are particularly grateful to Geraldine Jeffers and her team for their close support in getting this project underway. Our sincere thanks to Dennis Ola, Otto Mohr, and Alina Roser who provided constructive feedback on draft questions. Finally, profound thanks go to our families for their moral support and endless patience while we were writing this book.

CONTENTS

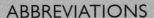

ABBREVIATIONS

ABPA	Allergic bronchopulmonary aspergillosis
ACE	Angiotensin-converting enzyme
ACTH	Adrenocorticotropic hormone
AD	Addison's disease
AED	Automated external defibrillator
AF	Atrial fibrillation
ALL	Acute lymphoblastic leukaemia
AML	Acute myeloblastic leukaemia
ANCA	Antineutrophil cytoplasmic antibodies
APTT	Activated partial thromboplastin time
ASA	American Society of Anesthesiologists
BAD	Bipolar affective disorder
BCR	Breakpoint cluster region
BMD	Bone mineral density
BMS	Burning mouth syndrome
BPH	Benign prostatic hyperplasia
BT	Bleeding time
CDT	Carbohydrate-deficient transferrin
CHHD	Clinical Human Health and Disease
CN	Cranial nerves
CNS	Central nervous system
COPD	Chronic obstructive pulmonary disease
CRP	C-reactive protein
CT	Computed tomography
DEXA	Dual-energy X-ray absorptiometry
DM	Diabetes mellitus
DMARD	Disease-modifying antirheumatic drug
DS	Down's syndrome
EMQs	Extended Matching Questions
ESR	Erythrocyte sedimentation rate
FBC	Full blood count

FNAC	Fine needle aspiration cytology
GABA	Gamma-aminobutyric acid
GCA	Giant cell arteritis
GDC	General Dental Council
GDP	General dental practitioner
GFR	Glomerular filtration rate
GGT	Gamma-glutamyl transpeptidase
GH	Growth hormone
GHRH	Growth hormone releasing hormone
GP	General practitioner
GVHD	Graft-versus-host disease
HDL	High density lipoprotein
HHD	Human Health and Disease
HHT	Hereditary haemorrhagic telangiectasia
HZ	Herpes zoster
IBD	Inflammatory bowel disease
IBS	Irritable bowel syndrome
ICU	Intensive care unit
INR	International normalized ratio
LCH	Langerhans cell histiocytosis
LDL	Low-density lipoprotein
MC	Microscopic colitis
MCV	Mean cell volume
MM	Multiple myeloma
MPNST	Malignant peripheral nerve sheath tumour
MRONJ	Medication-related osteonecrosis of the jaw
MRSA	Methicillin-resistant *Staphylococcus aureus*
MSH	Melanocyte-stimulating hormone
NBCCS	Naevoid basal cell carcinoma syndrome
NICE	National Institute for Clinical Excellence
NK	Natural killer
NSAID	Non-steroidal anti-inflammatory drugs
NSCLC	Non-small cell lung cancer
OCD	Obsessive-compulsive disorder
PCD	Primary ciliary dyskinesia
PEA	Pulseless electrical activity
PK	Pyruvate kinase
PTH	Parathyroid hormone
RAS	Renin-angiotensin system

RBC	Red blood cell
RPR	Rapid plasma reagin
SBA	Single best answer
TSC	Tuberous sclerosis complex
TSH	Thyroid-stimulating hormone
UK	United Kingdom
UKMI	UK Medicines Information
UMN	Upper motor neurone
VDRL	Venereal Disease Research Laboratory
VF	Ventricular fibrillation
VN	Virchow node
VT	Ventricular tachycardia
VZV	Varicella zoster virus

SINGLE BEST ANSWER (SBA) QUESTIONS

Introduction

Well-written single best answer (SBA) questions are currently held to be the format of choice for knowledge assessments in high stakes undergraduate and postgraduate examinations. They may also be useful adjunct to learning. In this chapter, each SBA consists of a clinical scenario, associated question, and a list of five plausible options. Of the five options, the MOST likely option is the correct answer, while the other four are incorrect options. In some of the more challenging SBAs one of the four incorrect answers may be partially correct but does not answer the question as well as the correct response.

Therapeutics in dentistry

1. **A mucous membrane pemphigoid patient on dapsone has developed massive red blood cell haemolysis, a known side effect. Which ONE of the following characteristic clinical features is this patient MOST likely to manifest?**
   A. Bradycardia
   B. Dark urine colour
   C. Lymphadenopathy
   D. Pale stool
   E. Spontaneous gingival bleeding

2. **A patient with atrial fibrillation and on warfarin is aware that certain drugs can interact with their medication to promote bleeding. Which ONE of the following drugs can be safely prescribed for dental treatment?**
   A. Erythromycin
   B. Metronidazole
   C. Miconazole
   D. Nystatin
   E. Tetracycline

3. **A 55-year-old patient is receiving prednisolone for polymyalgia rheumatica. Which ONE of the following advisories/information is MOST likely to be of benefit to this patient?**
   A. Advise adrenocortical suppression is unlikely
   B. Advise blood test to check triglyceride and potassium levels
   C. Advise an initial check of HB_{1Ac} at 6 months after commencing treatment
   D. Advise patient to avoid over the counter NSAID (non-steroidal anti-inflammatory drugs)
   E. Advise precautionary treatment for hypertension

4. **Post stem cell transplant for multiple myeloma, a patient is being placed on ciclosporin. Which ONE of the following is the MAIN side effect they may develop?**
   A. Nausea and vomiting
   B. Oral thrush
   C. Pancytopenia
   D. Recurrent oral ulcers
   E. Renal failure

5. **A patient with well-controlled hypertension presents with poor oral hygiene and generalized gum enlargement. Which ONE of the following antihypertensive medications is the MOST likely culprit?**
    A. Amlodipine
    B. Atenolol
    C. Bendroflumethiazide
    D. Losartan
    E. Ramipril

6. **You are about to prescribe an analgesic for post-extraction pain to a patient on prednisolone. Which ONE of the following analgesics can be SAFELY prescribed to this patient?**
    A. Aspirin
    B. Co-dydramol
    C. Diclofenac
    D. Mefenamic acid
    E. Paracetamol

7. **During a consultation you update a patient's drug history. The patient's medication includes ramipril, amlodipine, gliclazide, metformin, and simvastatin. Which ONE of the following options BEST describes the different classes of the patient's medication, respectively?**
    A. Angiotensin-converting enzyme inhibitor, calcium channel blocker, sulfonylurea, biguanide, and statins
    B. Angiotensin II receptor blocker, calcium channel blocker, alpha-glucosidase inhibitors biguanide, and statins
    C. Beta blocker, alpha blocker, sulfonylurea, biguanide, and statins
    D. Diuretic, calcium channel blocker, glitazone, sulfonyl urea, and statins
    E. Vasodilator, beta blocker, sulfonylurea, biguanide, and statins

8. **Lichenoid reaction is the histopathological diagnosis for a sore, white lacy-like lesion on the right buccal mucosa of a 60-year-old patient. In view of this finding, you have reviewed the patient's drug history with a view to identifying the possible causative medication. Which ONE of the following medications is MOST likely to be associated with the patient's oral finding?**
    A. Alendronic acid
    B. Bendroflumethiazide
    C. Co-codamol
    D. Pioglitazone
    E. Simvastatin

9. **A postmenopausal patient can't immediately recall a medication prescribed by the rheumatologists but remembers the instructions pertaining to it state** *'swallow the medicine with plenty of water before first meal or beverage of the day, remain upright for 30 minutes and wait 30 minutes before eating or using other drugs'*. **Which ONE of the following medicines is MOST likely been referred to?**

   A. Bisphosphonates
   B. Calcitonin
   C. Calcium and vitamin D supplements
   D. Hormone replacement therapy
   E. Strontium ranelate

10. **A patient presents with oral candidiasis (thrush). They are currently taking the following medications: atorvastatin, lansoprazole, ramipril, aspirin, metformin, and amlodipine. Which ONE of the following antifungals is MOST safe to prescribe to manage his thrush?**

    A. Fluconazole
    B. Itraconazole
    C. Miconazole
    D. Nystatin
    E. Terbinafine

11. **A patient on warfarin suffers from a recurrent infection at the angles of the mouth. They are using a prescribed medication for topical application. The international normalized ratio (INR) which was 2.8 now fluctuates between 3.7 and 4.5. Which one of the following is the MOST likely medication to cause this problem?**

    A. Betamethasone ointment
    B. Chlorhexidine gel
    C. Difflam mouthwash
    D. Miconazole gel
    E. Nystatin suspension

12. **A patient with hypertension and high blood cholesterol attends the emergency department with onset of increasingly severe muscular pain. Their medication includes** *daily simvastatin, aspirin, bendroflumethiazide,* **and** *clarithromycin* **which was prescribed 3 days ago for a spreading dentoalveolar abscess. Which ONE of the following tests below is MOST likely to be abnormal?**

    A. Raised alanine transaminase
    B. Raised alkaline phosphatase
    C. Raised creatinine kinase
    D. Raised lactate dehydrogenase
    E. Raised troponin

13. **Since commencing antibiotic treatment, a patient's INR readings has become raised and shown significant fluctuations. Their medical, drug, and allergy histories are as follows:**

Medical history—Atrial fibrillation
Drug history—Warfarin 5 mg daily
Allergy history—Penicillin

Which ONE of the following antibiotics is the MOST likely cause of the patient's raised and fluctuating INR reading?

A. Azithromycin
B. Cephalexin
C. Erythromycin
D. Trimethoprim
E. Vancomycin

Orofacial manifestations of systemic diseases

14. A young child who is seen regularly in the cardiac department, has learning difficulty, delayed tooth eruption, macroglossia, and characteristic facies. Which ONE of the following BEST describes the patient's findings?

A. Beckwith–Wiedemann syndrome
B. Cross syndrome
C. Down's syndrome
D. Myxoedema
E. Simpson–Golabi–Behmel syndrome

15. A patient presents with progressive dysphagia. On examination, there is pallor of the mucocutaneous tissues, and the tongue is denuded of the papilla. The resting pulse is fast and the nails on the hands and feet are either flat or concave in shape. Which ONE of the following syndromes is the MOST likely in this patient?

A. Gardner syndrome
B. Glanzmann's syndrome
C. Melkersson–Rosenthal syndrome
D. Peutz–Jeghers syndrome
E. Plummer–Vinson syndrome

16. A patient presents with a history of increasing obesity and depression. They have noticed a yellow tinge to the colour of their skin and increasing malaise. In addition, they have required their flat to remain heated throughout the year. Which ONE of the following oral manifestations is this patient MOST likely to develop?

A. Macroglossia
B. Median rhomboid glossitis
C. Recurrent oral ulcers
D. Spaced dentition
E. Spontaneous gingival bleeding

17. Skull imaging showed multiple discrete punched-out lesions. Blood tests show a raised erythrocyte sedimentation rate (ESR), hypercalcaemia, and abnormal plasma electrophoresis. Which ONE of the following is the MOST likely diagnosis for this patient?

A. Langerhans's histiocytosis
B. Metastatic bone disease
C. Multiple myeloma
D. Paget's disease of the bone
E. Secondary hyperparathyroidism

18. **A patient presents glossitis and peripheral sensory paraesthesia of hands and feet. They have had gastrectomy for management of gastric cancer. Which ONE of the following treatments are they MOST likely to benefit from?**
    A. Blood transfusion
    B. Intramuscular erythropoietin
    C. Intramuscular vitamin B_{12}
    D. Oral ferrous fumarate
    E. Oral hydroxocobalamin

19. **An overweight teenage girl presents with increasing amount of facial hair. She has a history of late onset of menstruation, secondary amenorrhoea, and recent onset of sleep apnoea. She is currently on metformin. Which ONE of the following is the MOST likely diagnosis for this patient?**
    A. Cushing's syndrome
    B. Hypogonadism
    C. Hypothyroidism
    D. Polycystic ovary syndrome
    E. Prolactinoma

20. **A patient presents to the orthodontist for treatment of a class III malocclusion. Examination reveals prominent supraorbital ridges and bitemporal hemianopia. Intraoral examination elicits increased spacing of the dentition and macroglossia. Which ONE of the following is the MOST likely cause of this patients' visual defect?**
    A. Craniopharyngioma
    B. Intracranial meningioma
    C. Neuroendocrine carcinoma
    D. Phaeochromocytoma
    E. Pituitary adenoma

21. **A child present with oral ulceration and abdominal pain. Examination reveals lip swelling, deep linear ulcers, mucosal tags, and unusual ridging of the buccal mucosa. Blood investigation revealed raised faecal calprotectin (elastase) and inflammatory markers. Which ONE of the following is MOST likely to be the diagnosis?**
    A. Coeliac disease
    B. Crohn's disease
    C. Irritable bowel syndrome
    D. Microscopic colitis
    E. Ulcerative colitis

22. **A patient with multiple maxillary bony exostosis is unable to have upper partial dentures fabricated. He has an annual colonoscopy to monitor intestinal polyps. Which ONE of the following eponymous syndromes BEST characterizes this patient's findings?**
    A. Gardner's syndrome
    B. Gorlin–Goltz syndrome
    C. Grinspan syndrome
    D. Melkersson–Rosenthal syndrome
    E. Peutz–Jeghers syndrome

23. **A teenage patient presents with multiple basal cell carcinoma-like lesions on the face. They are under review for bilateral odontogenic keratocysts at the maxillo-facial unit. Which ONE of the following eponymous syndromes BEST characterizes this patient's findings?**
    A. Albright syndrome
    B. Gardner syndrome
    C. Gorlin–Goltz syndrome
    D. Peutz–Jeghers syndrome
    E. Plummer–Vinson syndrome

24. **A patient with multiple telangiectatic spots on the lip and buccal mucosa experiences recurrent epistaxis and menorrhagia. Full blood count and peripheral smear revealed slightly low haemoglobin and microcytosis, respectively. Which ONE of the following eponymous syndromes BEST represents the patient's findings?**
    A. Angina bullosa haemorrhagia
    B. Bernard–Soulier syndrome
    C. Osler–Weber–Rendu syndrome
    D. Peutz–Jeghers syndrome
    E. Sturge–Weber syndrome

25. **A patient with multiple pigmented macules on the face and buccal mucosa is found to have polyps on colonoscopy. Which ONE of the following eponymous syndromes BEST represents the patient's findings?**
    A. Addison disease
    B. Gardener's syndrome
    C. Laugier–Hunziker–Baran syndrome
    D. Melkersson–Rosenthal syndrome
    E. Peutz–Jeghers syndrome

26. **A patient presents with multiple skin nodules and brown spots first noticed during childhood. The lesions have increased in size and number with age. Which ONE of the following conditions BEST fits with these skin manifestations?**
   A. Addison's disease
   B. Basal cell carcinoma
   C. Neurofibromatosis
   D. Peutz–Jeghers syndrome
   E. Tuberous sclerosis

27. **A young boy attends for routine dental review. He is found to have hypodontia with scant fine hair, no eyelashes and eyebrows, and dry skin. Which ONE of the following BEST characterizes this boy's orofacial presentations?**
   A. Down's syndrome
   B. Ectodermal dysplasia
   C. Ehlers–Danlos syndrome
   D. Fibrous dysplasia
   E. Pierre–Robinson syndrome

28. **A pregnant woman has a localized fleshy red gingival lump between the mandibular left first and second premolars. The lesion bleeds occasionally and first appeared during pregnancy. Which ONE of the following BEST characterizes the oral lesion?**
   A. Fibrous epulis
   B. Giant cell tumour
   C. Gingiva hypertrophy
   D. Pregnancy gingivitis
   E. Pyogenic granuloma

Haematological diseases

29. **A patient with a week's history of sore throat, fever, malaise, cervical lymphadenopathy, and palatal petechiae develops abdominal tenderness. Following an emergency computed tomography (CT) scan which showed an enlarged spleen, they underwent an urgent splenectomy. Which ONE of the following conditions is the MOST likely reason underlying the need for the patient's splenectomy?**
   A. Autoimmune haemolytic anaemia
   B. Felty's syndrome
   C. Infectious mononucleosis
   D. Sickle cell disease
   E. Thrombocytopenic purpura

30. **An elderly patient with atrial fibrillation has accidentally taken double their normal warfarin dose. Their INR is 9.6 and they have no obvious signs of bleeding. Which ONE of the following is MOST appropriate to manage this patient?**
   A. Stop warfarin and administer fresh frozen plasma
   B. Stop warfarin and administer oral vitamin K
   C. Stop warfarin and administer prothrombin complex concentrate
   D. Stop warfarin and administer recombinant factor VIIa
   E. Stop warfarin and monitor INR more frequently

31. **A patient on warfarin, simvastatin, ramipril, ibuprofen, and bendroflumethiazide requires a tooth extraction. Which ONE of the following special investigations SHOULD be requested before the extraction?**
   A. Activated partial thromboplastin time (APTT)
   B. Bleeding time (BT)
   C. Clotting factor assays
   D. Full blood count (FBC)
   E. Prothrombin time (PT)

32. **A patient with haemophilia attends for routine dental care complaining of spontaneous gingival bleeding since his last appointment. You suspect this may be caused by gingivitis. Which ONE of the following bleeding investigation or assays would be MOST appropriate in this circumstance?**
   A. Activated partial thromboplastin time (APTT)
   B. Bleeding time (BT)
   C. INR
   D. Prothrombin time (PT)
   E. Von Willebrand factor (vWF)

33. **A patient with hypertension and hypercholesterolemia is taking atenolol, amlodipine, simvastatin, and prophylactic aspirin daily and requires an emergency tooth extraction. Which ONE of the following steps is MOST appropriate to minimize post-extraction bleeding?**

A. Advise patient to stop aspirin 72 hours pre extraction then restart 48 hours post extraction

B. Advise patient to stop aspirin 24 hours preceding the extraction

C. Consult the patient's general medical practitioner via telephone before the extraction

D. Request the patient's INR

E. Suture the extraction socket and pack with an appropriate haemostatic agent

34. **A homeless alcoholic patient is seen in an emergency dental clinic complaining of recurrent oral ulceration and angular cheilitis. He started living rough about 1 year ago. He recently had a FBC undertaken through the general medical practitioner attached to his hostel. He has a copy of the results with him, reproduced in the following list (normal ranges are in parentheses):**

Haemoglobin—8 g/dl   [12–15 g/dl]
Red blood cell count—5.0×10^{12}/L   [4.5–6.5×10^{12}/L]
White blood cell count—7.0×10^{12}/L   [4.0–11.0×10^{12}/L]
Platelet count—250×10^{9}/L   [150–400×10^{12}/L]
Mean cell volume—125 fl   [80–100 fl]
Mean cell haemoglobin—27 pg   [27–32 pg]
Mean cell haemoglobin concentration—32 g/dl   [32–36 g/dl]
Peripheral blood smear—megaloblasts and hypersegmented neutrophils
Vitamin B_{12} assay—normal

Which ONE of the following combination of investigations is the MOST likely to be of diagnostic value?

A. Liver function test and ferritin

B. Liver function test and iron studies

C. Liver function test and serum folate

D. Liver function test and urea and electrolytes

E. Liver function test, magnesium, zinc, and serum B_{12}

35. **A patient with Crohn's disease who has had a complete ileectomy now has lip paraesthesia, recurrent soreness of the angles of the mouth and tongue. Which ONE of the following factors is MOST likely to account for the patient's oral manifestations?**

A. Diminished intrinsic factor production

B. Gastric parietal cell destruction

C. Malabsorption

D. Malnutrition

E. Pancreatic insufficiency

36. **A young African boy with sickle cell anaemia (SS) presents for routine dental evaluation. Which ONE of the following clinical features of SS and corresponding pathophysiological mechanisms BEST match?**

    A. Bone pain—Alveolar osteitis
    B. Gallstones—Increased unconjugated bilirubin in urine
    C. Glossitis—Vitamin B_{12} deficiency
    D. Jaundice—Glucose-6-phosphate dehydrogenase deficiency
    E. Maxillary prognathism—Erythroid hyperplasia

37. **A patient with active Crohn's disease is commenced on 40 mg prednisolone daily. He sees his gastroenterologist 4 weeks later and has a number of blood investigations including a FBC. Which ONE of the following blood findings is MOST likely to be associated with the patient's treatment?**

    A. Anaemia
    B. Granulocytopaenia
    C. Lymphocytosis
    D. Neutrophil leucocytosis
    E. Thrombocytopenia

38. **A 7-year-old child presents at the medical emergency department with spontaneous gingival bleeding, engorged gums, bilateral angular cheilitis, and thrush. An urgent FBC revealed low haemoglobin levels and a markedly raised white blood cell count. Which ONE of the following is the MOST likely diagnosis?**

    A. Acute lymphoblastic leukaemia
    B. Acute myeloblastic leukaemia
    C. Bone marrow failure
    D. Burkitt's lymphoma
    E. Chronic myeloid leukaemia

39. **A patient who is currently been investigated for recurrent epistaxis requires an urgent tooth extraction at the dental unit. Her most recent haemostatic screen in hospital is as follows (normal values in parentheses):**

Platelet count: 100×100^9/L   [150×100^9/L]
Bleeding time: Prolonged
INR: Normal
Von Willebrand Factor (vWF): Normal
Factor VIII: Normal
Factor IX: Normal

Which ONE of the following measures are you MOST likely to recommend to minimize post-extraction oozing?

A. Apply local haemostatic measures post extraction
B. Prescribe tranexamic acid mouth rinses post extraction
C. Proceed with the extraction as normal
D. Refer to hospital for platelet transfusion pre extraction
E. Refer to physician for a course of systemic corticosteroids pre extraction

40. **An elderly woman with Plummer–Vinson syndrome has regular follow-up visits to check for premalignant changes. Which ONE of the following is the MOST likely site where such changes can occur?**

A. Lip commissures
B. Nasopharynx
C. Post-cricoid areas
D. Retromolar areas
E. Tonsillar areas

41. **A 45-year-old patient with a history of weight loss, night sweats, fatigue, and neck lymph node enlargement has a lymph node biopsy. The biopsy displays a nodular architecture and occasional large Reed–Sternberg cells. Immunohistochemistry for EBER (Epstein–Barr virus [EBV] encoded RNA) is positive. Which ONE of the following is the MOST likely cause of the patient's neck lump?**

A. Burkitt's lymphoma
B. Diffuse large B-cell lymphoma
C. Hodgkin's lymphoma
D. Infectious mononucleosis
E. NK/T-cell lymphoma

Special investigations in relation to medicine in dentistry

42. **A 57-year-old man with bleeding gum, night sweat, fever, and lethargy is found to have 'Philadelphia chromosome' on genetic screening. Which ONE of the following haematological malignancies is this MOST likely to be indicative of?**
    A. Acute lymphoblastic leukaemia
    B. Burkitt's lymphoma
    C. Chronic lymphocytic leukaemia
    D. Chronic myeloid leukaemia
    E. Hodgkin's lymphoma

43. **A 54-year-old Afro-Caribbean patient with longstanding bronchiectasis has macroglossia. Chest radiography shows signs consistent with bronchial destruction. Tongue biopsy was positive for Congo-red stain under polarized light. Which ONE of the following is MOST likely to be the cause of the patient's macroglossia?**
    A. Acromegaly
    B. Amyloidosis
    C. Multiple myeloma
    D. Sarcoidosis
    E. Tuberculosis

44. **You are concerned that a 9-year-old boy with spontaneous gum bleeding, widespread oral thrush, and angular cheilitis may have a haematological malignancy. Which ONE of the following special investigations would be MOST helpful in establishing a definitive diagnosis?**
    A. Bone marrow biopsy
    B. Coagulation profile
    C. FBC with differential
    D. Peripheral blood smear
    E. Serum electrophoresis

45. **A patient with polydipsia, lethargy, depression, and abdominal pains has hypercalcaemia and a monoclonal light chain paraprotein band on special investigations. Which ONE of the following is the MOST likely cause of the patient's findings?**
    A. Bony metastases
    B. Hyperparathyroidism
    C. Multiple myeloma
    D. Paget's disease
    E. Sarcoidosis

46. Post thyroidectomy, a patient undergoes a number of clinical chemistry investigations which showed hypocalcaemia, hyperphosphatemia, and normal alkaline phosphatase levels. The patient also has circumoral paraesthesia and spasms. Which ONE of the following is the MOST likely cause of the patient's findings?

A. Hypomagnesaemia

B. Hypoparathyroidism

C. Hypothyroidism

D. Postoperative critical illness

E. Vitamin D deficiency

47. An obese woman with lethargy, flat affect, low mood, and cold intolerance has yellowish plaque deposits around her eye lids. Which ONE of the following findings is MOST likely on special investigation?

A. Decreased high density lipoprotein (HDL) and low thyroxine (T4) levels

B. Decreased low density lipoprotein (LDL) and low thyroxine (T4) levels

C. Increased HDL and low thyroid-stimulating hormone (TSH) levels

D. Increased LDL and low TSH levels

E. Increased LDL and low thyroxine (T4) levels

48. A man presents with lethargy, abdominal pain, nausea, and vomiting and hyperpigmentation of the skin and mouth. He is been urgently referred to the endocrinologist. Which ONE of the following special investigations is MOST helpful in establishing the underlying cause of the patient's findings?

A. Adrenocorticotropic hormone (ACTH) stimulation test

B. Dexamethasone suppression test

C. Serum aldosterone and renin levels

D. Serum cortisol level

E. Serum electrolyte levels

49. A thin post-menopausal Asian woman who smokes 10 cigarettes daily requires prednisolone to treat pemphigus vulgaris. Which ONE of the following special investigations is MOST important for routine monitoring in this patient?

A. Bone mineral density measurement by DEXA scan

B. Bone mineral density measurement by quantitative ultrasound of the heel

C. Bone mineral density measurement by X-ray of the hips, wrists, and spine

D. Bone profile blood test

E. Hormone prolife blood test

50. **A facial nerve examination in a patient with end-stage kidney disease and vitamin D deficiency elicited spasm of the facial muscles. Which ONE of the following signs BEST describes this examination finding?**

A. Battle's sign

B. Chvostek's sign

C. Nikolsky's sign

D. Russell's sign

E. Trousseau's sign

Medical emergencies in dentistry

51. **A patient taking long-term prednisolone collapses during dental treatment. He is breathing but has a reduced level of consciousness. Which ONE of the following steps is the MOST important one in the initial management of this patient?**
    A. Administer oxygen and 1 mg of glucagon intramuscularly when fully conscious
    B. Administer oxygen and discharge when fully conscious
    C. Administer oxygen and oral glucose
    D. Administer oxygen and place patient in the recovery position
    E. Administer oxygen with the patient laid flat and call the ambulance services

52. **An elderly patient on pravastatin, bisoprolol, amlodipine, and bendroflumethiazide experiences transient episodes of light-headedness after standing up. Which ONE of the following is the MOST likely condition the patient is experiencing?**
    A. Hypoglycaemia
    B. Orthostatic hypotension
    C. Pseudo-syncope
    D. Vasovagal syncope
    E. Vertigo

53. **Post administration of parenteral penicillin, a patient becomes pale, clammy, dizzy, and short of breath. He also develops hives and patchy erythematous areas on his skin. Which ONE of the following classes of medication is the MOST important to manage the patient's medical emergency?**
    A. Antihistamines
    B. Catecholamines
    C. Corticosteroids
    D. Oxygen
    E. β_2 agonists

54. **An asthmatic patient has developed shortness of breath and breathing difficulty after using naproxen for post-extraction pain. Which ONE of the following findings in the patient's medical history is the MOST useful in predicting the risk of developing the patient's medical emergency?**
    A. History of daily use of inhaled corticosteroids
    B. History of food allergy
    C. History of ongoing upper respiratory tract infection
    D. History of parental atopy
    E. History of use of one salbutamol inhaler canister in the preceding 3 months

55. **An elderly patient develops slurred speech, saliva drooling, facial drooping, and arm weakness on the left-side and is confused. Which ONE of the following findings in the patient's history is MOST likely to be aetiologically associated with this patient's medical emergency?**
   A. Atrial fibrillation
   B. Hypothyroidism
   C. NSAIDs use
   D. Oral contraceptive use
   E. Sickle cell disease

56. **A new dental nurse has been provided the practice policy for management of medical emergencies. Which ONE of the following options MOST reflect current practice as determined by the Resuscitation council?**
   A. Medical emergency drugs and equipment must be safely stored in a secured place
   B. Medical emergency drugs excluding oxygen should only be given by dentists
   C. Medical history should only be obtained from new patients
   D. Resuscitation equipment (including AED) and emergency drugs must be checked monthly
   E. Resuscitation training is mandatory for only dentists

57. **A 75-year-old male patient reports occasional episodes of light-headedness when standing for prolonged periods. His medical history includes type 2 diabetes and benign prostatic hypertrophy. Which ONE of the following medications is MOST likely to cause the patient's symptoms?**
   A. Aspirin
   B. Clopidogrel
   C. Metformin
   D. Simvastatin
   E. Tamsulosin

58. **You suspect a patient may have experienced a cerebrovascular accident (CVA). Which ONE of the following clinical features is MOST likely in a CVA?**
   A. Drooping angle of the mouth
   B. Furrowing of the brow
   C. Hyperacusis
   D. Loss of blink reflex
   E. Painful rash over the ear

59. **A patient has recovered from an epileptic seizure in your practice. In which ONE of the following scenarios is calling the emergency helpline '999' recommended?**
   A. History of convulsive episodes lasting no more than 5 minutes
   B. History of more than three episodes of jerking movements of the limb in an hour
   C. History of seizures episodes but with good control
   D. Patient experienced frothing from the mouth and post-ictal incontinence
   E. Patient is conscious but breathing is noisy

60. **In which ONE of the following medical emergencies is calling the emergency helpline '999' and transfer to hospital an absolute requirement irrespective of recovery following initial management?**
   A. Anaphylactic attack
   B. Asthmatic attack
   C. Epileptic attack
   D. Hypoglycaemic attack
   E. Syncopal attack

Rheumatological diseases

61. **A 55-year-old patient with pain and tender scalp and jaw claudication on the same side is immediately referred to the emergency department. Special investigations revealed raised ESR. Which ONE of the following is the MOST likely cause of her symptoms?**
    A. Polymyalgia rheumatica
    B. Polymyositis
    C. Takayasu's arteritis
    D. Temporal arteritis
    E. Trigeminal neuralgia

62. **A patient with Paget's disease of the bone treated with intravenous bisphosphonates attends your practice for a routine appointment. Which ONE of the following are you MOST concerned about in this patient?**
    A. Bone pain
    B. Hearing loss
    C. Muscle pain
    D. Osteonecrosis
    E. Osteosarcoma

63. **A patient with oral graft versus host disease and on azathioprine, prednisolone, and acyclovir reports episodes of acute back pain on sitting and standing which is relieved by bed rest. Which ONE of the following is the MOST likely cause of the patient's back pain?**
    A. Osteoarthritis
    B. Osteodystrophy
    C. Osteomalacia
    D. Osteomyelitis
    E. Osteoporosis

64. **A patient with hearing loss has difficulty wearing a recently made upper denture. Blood tests showed a markedly raised bone derived alkaline phosphatase, normal serum calcium, phosphate, and 25-hydroxyvitamin D. Which ONE of the following is the MOST likely cause of the patient's findings?**
    A. Acromegaly
    B. Osteomalacia
    C. Osteoporosis
    D. Osteosarcoma
    E. Paget's disease

65. You are uncertain if a patient with prominent supraorbital ridges and macroglossia may have acromegaly. Which **ONE** of the following is the **MOST** reliable marker to establish the diagnosis following blood tests?

A. Serum calcium
B. Serum glucose
C. Serum growth hormone
D. Serum insulin-like growth factor 1
E. Serum phosphate

66. A new resident who became acutely unwell and confused has suffered a fracture of the neck of femur following a fall at a care home. Which **ONE** of the following factors is **MOST** likely to have contributed to the patient's fracture?

A. Delirium
B. Dementia
C. Depression
D. Polypharmacy
E. Poor diet

67. A 42-year-old female model has a fall resulting in a fracture and is diagnosed with osteoporosis. Which **ONE** of the following diets is **MOST** likely to have contributed to the development of her osteoporosis?

A. Gluten-free diet
B. Macrobiotic diet
C. Paleo diet
D. Vegan diet
E. Vegetarian diet

68. A patient is prescribed emergency prednisolone for temporal tenderness and visual symptoms. The doctor is concerned the patient could become blind if left untreated. Which **ONE** of the following **BEST** represents the patient condition?

A. Fibromyalgia
B. Giant cell arteritis
C. Polyarteritis nodosa
D. Polymyalgia rheumatica
E. Takayasu's arteritis

Cardiac diseases

69. **Having updated a patient's medication history, the list includes rivaroxaban, atenolol, simvastatin, and amiodarone for management of a cardiac arrhythmia. Which ONE of the following is the MOST likely cardiac arrhythmia being managed?**
    A. Atrial fibrillation
    B. Atrial flutter
    C. Sinus bradycardia
    D. Sinus tachycardia
    E. Ventricular tachycardia

70. **A patient with hypertension cannot remember the name of their medication; fortunately, they have brought with them the drug pack which is labelled 'Losartan, Take ONE daily'. Which ONE of the following classes of antihypertensive drugs does losartan belong to?**
    A. Angiotensin II receptor antagonist
    B. Angiotensin-converting enzyme inhibitors
    C. Beta blocker
    D. Loop diuretic
    E. Thiazide diuretic

71. **A 29-year-old patient with angina has bilateral corneal arcus and yellow lesions at the inner canthus of the eye and on the eyelids. Which ONE of the following is the MOST likely diagnostic inference to be drawn from these facial findings?**
    A. Cushing's syndrome
    B. Familial hypercholesterolaemia
    C. Hypothyroidism
    D. Nephrotic syndrome
    E. Obstructive jaundice

72. **A patient with a history of cardiovascular disease is on the following medications: indapamide, bisoprolol, and amlodipine. Which ONE of the following BEST represents the class of each drug, respectively?**
    A. Aldosterone antagonist, β-adrenergic receptor blocker, and calcium channel blocker
    B. Loop diuretic, β-adrenergic receptor blocker, and potassium channel blockers
    C. Osmotic diuretic, α-adrenergic receptor blocker, and β-adrenergic receptor blocker
    D. Potassium sparing diuretic, α-adrenergic receptor blocker, and calcium channel blocker
    E. Thiazide-like diuretic, β-adrenergic receptor blocker, and calcium channel blocker

73. An automatic external defibrillator detects a rhythm which necessitates defibrillation during basic life support for a patient with a cardiac arrest. Which ONE of the following rhythms is MOST likely to represents this patient cardiac rhythm?

A. Asystole

B. Pulseless electrical activity

C. Pulseless ventricular tachycardia

D. Sinus tachycardia

E. Supraventricular tachycardia

74. A patient on dabigatran to manage atrial fibrillation requires surgical extraction of an unerupted lower third molar. Which ONE of the following is the MOST appropriate precautions to be taken to minimize the risk of post-extraction bleeding?

A. Administer vitamin K, preoperatively

B. Advise patient to miss morning dose on the extraction day and when to restart

C. Apply local haemostatic measures and sutures to manage bleeding postoperatively

D. Ensure the patient's APTT is checked no more than 24 hours before the extraction

E. Ensure the patient's INR is checked no more than 24 hours before the extraction

Neurological diseases

75. **A patient with a malignant parotid swelling presents with a facial palsy. Which ONE of the following cranial nerves (CN) is the MOST likely to be involved?**

    A. III
    B. V
    C. VI
    D. VII
    E. VIII

76. **A 70-year-old patient with a lower midline neck swelling presents hoarseness of voice, difficulty in breathing, weight loss, and malaise. On examination, the swelling is ill-defined, hard, and moves on protrusion of the tongue. Which ONE of the following is the MOST likely cause of the patient's neck swelling?**

    A. Adenomatoid nodule
    B. Follicular adenoma
    C. Multinodular goitre
    D. Papillary thyroid carcinoma
    E. Undifferentiated carcinoma

77. **A patient with herpes zoster ophthalmicus presents with severe pain and vesicles around the left eye. Which ONE of the following is MOST likely to be associated with this condition?**

    A. Dermatome involvement
    B. External auditory canal rash
    C. Facial paralysis
    D. Follicular type mucocutaneous eruptions
    E. Rash extending across the forehead midline

78. **A young child with convergent squint in the left eye experiences double vision on lateral gaze. Which ONE of the following CN is the MOST likely affected?**

    A. III
    B. IV
    C. V
    D. VI
    E. VII

79. **The left eye of a patient with multiple sclerosis deviates down and out on forward gaze. On examination, lid droop and dilated unreactive pupil are noted. Which ONE of the following is the MOST likely affected cranial nerve?**

    A. II
    B. III
    C. IV
    D. VI
    E. VII

Endocrine diseases

80. **A general practitioner (GP) refers a thin patient with bulging eyes, excessive sweating, and heat intolerance for an electrocardiography (ECG) to determine if they have an arrhythmia. Which ONE of the following cardiac arrhythmias is MOST likely to be detected in this patient?**
    A. Atrial flutter
    B. Sinus bradycardia
    C. Sinus tachycardia
    D. Ventricular fibrillation
    E. Ventricular tachycardia

81. **A general dental practitioner (GDP) noticed periorbital puffiness and loss of the outer third of the eyebrows in a patient who attends dental review regularly. Enquiries about the patient's general health revealed tiredness, lack of motivation, and recent weight gain. The patient attends her GP and autoantibody testing was subsequently found to be positive. Which ONE of the following autoantibodies is MOST likely to be detected in this patient?**
    A. 21-hydroxylase
    B. Acetyl choline receptor
    C. Intrinsic factor
    D. Thyroglobulin and thyroid peroxidase
    E. TSH receptor

82. **A patient with diffuse and bilateral oral hyperpigmentation has persistent low blood pressure at checks during routine dental reviews. Which ONE of the following is the MOST likely cause of the patient's findings?**
    A. Addison's disease
    B. Conn's syndrome
    C. Cowden disease
    D. Cushing's syndrome
    E. Peutz–Jeghers syndrome

83. **A diabetic patient taking oral hypoglycaemic drugs presents multiple periodontal abscesses at a recent dental review. The patient's GP has requested an Hb$_{1Ac}$ blood test to ascertain why. Which ONE of the following BEST depicts what Hb$_{1Ac}$ measures?**

    A. Cumulative blood glucose in preceding 3 months
    B. Cumulative blood glucose in preceding 3 weeks
    C. Long-term measure of fasting blood glucose
    D. Longitudinal measure of random blood glucose
    E. Random blood ketones

Infectious diseases

84. A patient has developed jaundice, headache, and malaise on return from a trip to Zanzibar. Blood tests showed normocytic anaemia, reticulocytosis, and a raised unconjugated bilirubin level. Which ONE of the following is the MOST likely cause of the patient's findings?
    A. Glucose-6-phosphate dehydrogenase deficiency
    B. Malaria
    C. Pyruvate kinase deficiency
    D. Sickle cell disease
    E. Spherocytosis

85. A patient presents cervical lymphadenopathy and a painless firm tongue ulcer. They have also had a genital ulcer which has completely healed after 4 weeks. You suspect this patient may have syphilis. Which ONE of the following investigations is MOST likely to be of diagnostic value in this patient?
    A. Dark field microscopy
    B. Gram staining
    C. Microbiology and culture
    D. Polymerase chain reaction
    E. Rapid plasma reagin

86. A teenage patient presents fever, malaise, and sore throat. On examination they have bilateral cervical lymphadenopathy and palatal petechiae. A monospot's test was remarkable. Which ONE of the following viruses is MOST likely to be the cause of the patient's findings?
    A. Coxsackie virus
    B. Cytomegalovirus
    C. Epstein–Barr virus
    D. Herpes virus
    E. Herpes zoster virus

87. A patient with a non-healing tongue ulcer and cervical lymphadenopathy presents night sweats, weight loss, and nocturnal fever. Biopsy of the ulcer showed necrotizing granulomas. Which ONE of the following is the MOST likely cause of the patient's oral findings?
    A. Actinomycosis
    B. Granulomatosis with polyangiitis (Wegener's granulomatosis)
    C. Orofacial granulomatosis
    D. Sarcoidosis
    E. Tuberculosis

Psychiatry in dentistry

88. **A longstanding work colleague has previously suffered from profound depression but recently you have noticed that he has become excessively cheerful (often inappropriately so) and at times irritable and aggressive. His partner confides in you that he is hardly sleeping. This behaviour is beginning to affect his work and you wonder if he is having a manic episode as part of bipolar affective disorder. Which ONE of the following clinical features would be most consistent with this diagnosis?**
    A. Delusions of personal inadequacy
    B. Fatigue and loss of energy
    C. Inappropriate sexual encounters
    D. Reduced pleasure in normally pleasurable activities
    E. Weight gain

89. **In addition to brushing teeth many times each day, a young patient rinses her mouth with mouthwash as many as 20 times daily. She is convinced that she has oral malodour despite repeated reassurances from her dentist and specialists. Which ONE of the following diagnoses BEST characterizes the patient's behaviour?**
    A. Depression
    B. Generalized anxiety disorder
    C. Hypochondriasis
    D. Obsessive-compulsive disorder
    E. Paranoid personality disorder

90. **Over the past 2 months the previously cheerful practice receptionist has appeared less energetic and quieter than previously. He appears to have lost weight and you are concerned about his health. When you ask him how he's doing he reports that he's been 'feeling very low'. Which ONE of the following symptoms would be MOST consistent with a diagnosis of depression?**
    A. Auditory hallucinations involving a running commentary on his behaviour
    B. Cold intolerance
    C. Disorientation for time
    D. Reduced interest or enjoyment in previously pleasurable activities
    E. Thought broadcasting, echo, insertion, or withdrawal

91. **A patient appears disoriented, sweaty, and clammy after having a local anaesthetic injection. They are breathing rapidly and have an intense tingling sensation around their mouth. They complain of palpitations and chest pain. Without intervention, the symptoms resolve after 10 minutes. Which ONE of the following is the MOST likely cause of the patient's findings?**
    A. Anaphylactic attack
    B. Asthmatic attack
    C. Epileptic attack
    D. Panic attack
    E. Syncopal attack

92. **A patient attends their dental appointment after cancelling or missing a number of previous appointments. They are currently going through a divorce and say that they feel like 'ending it all'. Which ONE of the following factors is MOST likely to prevent this patient from attempting suicide?**
    A. Alcohol abuse
    B. Clinical depression
    C. Family support
    D. Healthcare worker
    E. Previous failed suicide attempt

93. **A patient with poorly controlled schizophrenia attends your dental practice complaining of toothache. While assessing the patient he starts talking to non-existent people who he claims he can hear discussing his dental problems. Which ONE of the following descriptive terms BEST describes this particular psychiatric symptom?**
    A. Delusion
    B. Hallucination
    C. Illusion
    D. Obsession
    E. Thought insertion

Immunological diseases

94. A young child present with itchy and generalized dryness of skin. Lately, the child has developed a hypopigmented patches on the face. A history of seasonal hay fever is noted in the medical history. Which ONE of the following immunoglobulins is MOST likely to be out of range?

A. IgA
B. IgD
C. IgE
D. IgG
E. IgM

95. A patient develops a rapid and marked swelling around the eyes and lips without any obvious triggers. In the past, they have had breathing difficulty which necessitated hospital care. Blood tests revealed low C1 esterase inhibitor (C-INH) levels. Which ONE of the following is the MOST likely to be associated with the patient's swellings?

A. Acquired angioedema
B. Allergic angioedema
C. Angiotensin-converting enzyme inhibitor (ACEi) induced angioedema
D. Hereditary angioedema
E. Idiopathic angioedema

Hand manifestations of systemic diseases

96. **A patient with a history of alcohol and substance misuse has been diagnosed with liver cirrhosis. Which ONE of the following finger/nail changes is MOST likely in this patient?**
    A. Beau's lines
    B. Finger clubbing
    C. Koilonychia
    D. Paronychia
    E. Splinter haemorrhages

97. **A patient with Plummer–Vinson syndrome is attending for regular dental review. Which ONE of the following nail abnormalities is this patient MOST likely to feature?**
    A. Brown little streak under the nails
    B. Indented spoon-shaped nails
    C. Pitting/dents on the nails
    D. Transverse groves across the nails
    E. White nails with reddened or dark tips

Gastrointestinal diseases

98. A young child presents mouth ulcers, tummy ache, bloating, and tiredness. Special tests showed raised faecal calprotectin and antiendomysial antibodies. Which ONE of the following is the MOST likely cause of the patient's features?
    A. Coeliac disease
    B. Crohn's disease
    C. Irritable bowel syndrome
    D. Symptomatic diverticular disease
    E. Ulcerative colitis

99. An elderly patient presents epigastric pain, weight loss, and malaise. On examination, an enlarged and fixed lymph node was palpated in the left supraclavicular fossa. Which ONE of the following was traditionally associated with the patient's physical findings?
    A. Breast carcinoma
    B. Bronchogenic carcinoma
    C. Colonic adenocarcinoma
    D. Gastric adenocarcinoma
    E. Hodgkin's lymphoma

100. An unkempt patient presents to Accident and Emergency after sustaining a head injury. The assessing Oral Surgery Registrar finds evidence of dental neglect with marked tooth surface loss and notices a heavy smell of alcohol. The registrar is concerned that the patient is an alcoholic. Which ONE of the following blood investigation results is MOST suggestive of excessive alcohol intake?
    A. Raised alanine transaminase (ALT)
    B. Raised aspartate transaminase (AST)
    C. Raised gamma-glutamyl transpeptidase (GGT)
    D. Raised mean cell volume (MCV)
    E. Raised megakaryocyte count

Renal diseases

101. A young child presents with a puffy face and swollen ankles. Urine test showed markedly raised protein levels. Which **ONE** of the following is the **MOST** likely diagnosis of the patient's findings?
   A. Interstitial nephritis
   B. Nephritic syndrome
   C. Nephrotic syndrome
   D. Polycystic kidney disease
   E. Urinary tract infection

102. A patient with end-stage renal disease from hypertensive nephrosclerosis has been on dialysis for several years. Which **ONE** of the following complications in this patient and corresponding pathophysiological mechanism **BEST** match?
   A. Bone pain—Reduced parathyroid hormone
   B. Brown tumour—Secondary hyperparathyroidism
   C. Hypertension—Raised parasympathetic stimulation
   D. Normocytic anaemia—Impaired haematinic utilization
   E. Prolonged bleeding—Raised platelet thromboxane

Respiratory diseases

103. An asthmatic patient on prophylactic steroid inhaler has recurrent oral thrush. He has been recommended a spacer device to alleviate his symptoms. Which **ONE** of the following statements **BEST** represents the benefits of a spacer device for this patient?

A. Reduced impact of hand-breath coordination problems

B. Reduced oropharyngeal deposition of steroid

C. Reduced requirement for good manual dexterity is the sole benefit for its use

D. Reduced respirable aerosol fraction of steroid due to electrostatic charge

E. Reduced systemic bioavailability of steroid but can be bulky device to use

104. A 65-year old man attends his GP surgery having been troubled by a worsening, nagging cough with occasional blood-stained sputum over the past 8 weeks. He has noticed progressive loss of appetite and weight loss. He is a lifelong cigarette smoker with a 35-year pack history. On examination he has axillary lymphadenopathy and finger clubbing. Which **ONE** of the following is the **MOST** likely diagnosis of this patient's findings?

A. Bronchiectasis

B. Exacerbation of chronic obstructive pulmonary disease

C. Lung cancer

D. Pulmonary embolism

E. Pulmonary oedema

105. A 30-year old patient attends for a routine dental appointment for the first time. The medical history is suggestive of severe asthma. Which **ONE** of the following history findings would be **MOST** indicative of the severity of this patient's asthma?

A. Concurrent use of two different types of asthma medication

B. Exacerbation of asthma by exercise

C. Hospital admission for breathlessness during the last year

D. Morning dips in peak expiratory flow rate

E. Sensitivity to paracetamol

106. **A 20-year-old with known asthma is having a routine dental procedure undertaken using local anaesthetic when she is noticed to be becoming increasingly wheezy. Which ONE of the following clinical symptoms and signs is MOST likely to suggest a respiratory arrest is imminent?**

  A. Loud wheeze throughout inhalation and exhalation
  B. Paradoxical thoracoabdominal movement
  C. Tachycardia
  D. Tachypnoea
  E. Talking in words

107. **A 50-year-old patient attending for routine dental treatment informs you that he has just been diagnosed as having 'asthma'. You wonder if he actually has chronic obstructive pulmonary disease (COPD). Which ONE of the following clinical features suggests that the patient is most likely to have COPD?**

  A. Chronic, productive cough
  B. Night-time wheeze
  C. No history of smoking
  D. Symptoms first occurred in childhood
  E. Variable severity of breathlessness

Preoperative anaesthetic care

108. A patient with dental phobia has opted for wisdom tooth extractions under general anaesthesia as a day-case surgery. Which ONE of the following preoperative findings is MOST likely to make this patient unsuitable for the extractions as a day-case surgery?

A. Angina at rest

B. Controlled type II diabetes mellitus

C. Has a responsible adult to escort and look after them at home

D. Obesity

E. Travelling time of less than 1 hour to the hospital

SBA ANSWERS, RATIONALE, AND FURTHER READING

Introduction

Answers, feedback, and explanations demonstrating why the correct answer is most plausible and other options are incorrect are provided in this chapter. Sign-posting to other sources of further information such as *Oxford Handbooks*, websites, and journal articles is also provided in this chapter.

Therapeutics in dentistry

1. B

Drug-induced immune haemolytic anaemia can be caused by many drugs including dapsone. The drugs bind covalently to proteins on the red blood cell (RBC) membrane such that circulating RBCs are heavily coated with the medication. This does no harm to the RBCs, however if a patient has IgG antibody to the medication (i.e. sensitized), the antibody will bind to the drug on the RBC. This will cause the RBCs to be recognized and phagocytized by the macrophage-monocyte system of the liver or spleen leading to FC-mediated extravascular RBC destruction; complement (C3b) may also be involved via opsonization. This drug-induced RBC destruction is an exacerbation of the physiologic process utilized to eliminate senescent circulating RBCs. Under normal circumstances, the lysed RBC releases it globin and iron which are recycled into amino acid pool and bound to transferrin respectively. Haem is broken down into protoporphyrin, then bilirubin, which is conjugated (made water soluble) in the liver. The conjugated bilirubin is converted into urobilinogen and stercobilinogen, both of which are excreted in urine and faeces, respectively. Both product impacts colour to urine and faeces. Where there is massive haemolysis of RBCs induced by dapsone, there is bilirubin overproduction (hyperbilirubinaemia), overwhelming the liver such that excessive unconjugated bilirubin sips into soft tissue manifesting as jaundice (yellowing of the skin, mucous membrane). The unconjugated bilirubinaemia in blood is filtered through the kidney and excessive urobilinogen produced impacts a dark colour to urine. The same applies for stool, in this case excessive stercobilinogen, a product of bilirubin conjugation also causes stool to have a darker appearance.

In summary, dapsone can cause prehepatic jaundice induced by haemolytic anaemia. The ensuing hyperbilirubinaemia can occur in all patients but more often in patients with glucose 6 phosphate dehydrogenase (G6PD) deficiency.

Other side effects of dapsone include isolated abnormalities of liver function tests, toxic or cholestatic hepatitis in conjunction with hypersensitivity syndrome, peripheral neuropathy, methaemoglobinaemia, headaches, photosensitivity, agranulocytosis, and hypersensitivity syndrome. Lymphadenopathy, fever, rash, hepatic dysfunction, leucocytosis, eosinophilia, and anaemia can occur as part of hypersensitivity syndrome.

With this background, pale stool, bradycardia, and spontaneous gingival bleeding are not plausible and therefore incorrect options. Lymphadenopathy and dark urine are both potential side effects. However, in view of the rarity of hypersensitivity syndrome of which lymphadenopathy is a clinical feature, the most likely option is dark urine.

Note: While prescription of dapsone is not within the remits of a general dental practitioner (GDP), it is likely you may come across a patient on dapsone therapy. For this reason it is important to know that prior to dapsone administration patients need to undergo a careful clinical evaluation which includes a thorough clinical history and physical examination and baseline routine blood investigations (i.e. full blood count with differentials, urinalysis, liver and renal function test, serology for hepatitis and G6PD levels). Post commencement of dapsone therapy, follow-up visits which include a good clinical history and regular repeat blood investigations as just highlighted are important to evaluate response to treatment and assess for potential adverse effects.

Further reading

Wozel G, Blasum C. Dapsone in dermatology and beyond. *Arch Dermatol Res*, 2014;306(2):103–24.

2. D

Various drug-metabolizing isoenzymes are involved with drug biotransformation, the most common being cytochrome CYP450. These enzymes can either be inhibited or induced by certain drugs. For example, rifampicin, induces CYP450, leading to increased metabolism, and clearance of the oral contraceptive pill resulting an unwanted pregnancy. In contrast, erythromycin, metronidazole, miconazole, and tetracycline block or inhibit CYP450, required for warfarin metabolism. Consequently, warfarin remains in its active form for longer in systemic circulation together with reduced drug clearance. Both effects result in a raised international normalized ratio (INR) and a significantly increased risk of bleeding.

Specifically, miconazole (Daktarin gel) when concomitantly used with warfarin is reported to enhance its anticoagulant effect by up to fivefold. Therefore, a patient on warfarin for AF is best not prescribed miconazole if indicated; but nystatin, a polyene antifungal, can be safely used.

Further reading

Dawoud BE, Roberts A, Yates JM. Drug interactions in general dental practice—considerations for the dental practitioner. *Br Dent J*, 2014;216:15–23.

3. D

One notable side effect of corticosteroids is the increase in gastric acid production in the stomach. Therefore, patients on corticosteroids are advised to avoid using over-the-counter medications like aspirin, non-steroidal anti-inflammatory drugs (NSAIDs), and ibuprofen because of an increased risk of developing duodenal ulcers/peptic ulceration. Other side effects include hypertension, weight gain, osteoporosis, growth suppression in children, raised triglycerides and potassium levels, adrenocortical suppression, and increased risk of developing glaucoma and cataracts. It is essential that baseline measurements are taken before starting treatment with steroids. During treatment patients should be regularly monitored, as outlined in Table 2.1.

Table 2.1 Side effects of corticosteroids and monitoring/precautionary steps instituted for prevention

Side effects	Monitoring/Precaution
Blood pressure	Monitor blood pressure regularly
Weight gain	Monitor body weight regularly
Growth suppression	Record height of children and adolescents regularly on a growth chart
Triglycerides and potassium	Check bloods for raised triglycerides and hypokalaemia, 1 month after initiating oral corticosteroids, then every 6–12 months thereafter
Hb_{A1c}	Check 1 month after initiation of oral corticosteroids, and every 3 months thereafter
Osteoporosis	Arrange for DEXA scan for people with pre-existing risk of osteoporosis
Adrenocortical suppression	Monitor for signs of adrenal suppression. During withdrawal, the dose of oral corticosteroids may be reduced rapidly down to physiological doses (about 7.5 mg of prednisolone or equivalent) and reduced more slowly thereafter

Further reading

National Institute for Health and Care Excellence. *Corticosteroids—Oral: Summary*, June 2020. Available at: https://cks.nice.org.uk/corticosteroids-oral#!topicSummary

4. E

Ciclosporin, an immunosuppressant drug, is a calcineurin inhibitor used for prevention and treatment of graft-versus-host disease following renal and other solid organ transplants. It selectively inhibits adaptive immune responses by blocking T-cell-dependent biosynthesis of lymphokines, particularly interleukin 2 at the level of messenger ribonucleic acid (mRNA) transcription.

Nausea and vomiting, oral thrush, pancytopenia, recurrent oral ulcers are possible but not the main side effects of ciclosporin; therefore not plausible options. The **MAIN** side effect of ciclosporin is renal failure, and therefore the correct option. The renal failure is a consequence of acute and chronic nephrotoxicity. The acute nephrotoxicity is thought to be due to vascular dysfunction, i.e. preferential constriction of the afferent renal arteriole induced by an increase in the vasoconstrictor factors endothelin, thromboxane as well as activation of the renin-angiotensin system (RAS). Simultaneously, there is a reduction in the vasodilator factors, prostacyclin, prostaglandin E2, and nitric oxide. In other words, there is an imbalance in vasoconstrictor and vasodilator factors which leads to significant reduction in renal blood flow and a rise in renal vascular resistance. The chronic nephrotoxicity is due to arteriolar hyalinosis and interstitial or so-called striped fibrosis, both of which will result in significant reductions in glomerular filtration rate (GFR), renal plasma flow, and renal blood flow.

Other well-known side effects of ciclosporin include hypertension, hyperlipidaemia, gingival hyperplasia, hyperkalaemia, neurotoxicity, hypomagnesaemia, hyperuricaemia, and thrombotic microangiopathy. These effects are thought in part due to calcineurin inhibition in non-lymphatic tissues.

Further reading

National Institute for Health and Care Excellence. *Ciclosporin.* Available at: https://bnf.nice.org.uk/drug/ciclosporin.html#sideEffects

5. A

The causes of gingival hyperplasia or hypertrophy can be broadly categorized into four groups. They include:

I. Inflammatory gingival enlargement
- **Causes**—Localized or generalized due to plaque accumulation.
- **Clinical features**—The gingiva is usually tender, soft, red, and bleed easily.
- **Management**—Improve oral hygiene practices.

II. Medication-induced gingival enlargement
- **Causes**—Associated with certain medications, the most commonly implicated include phenytoin, ciclosporin and calcium channel blockers (e.g. verapamil, felodipine, lacidipine, lercanidipine hydrochloride, nicardipine hydrochloride, nifedipine, and nimodipine).
- **Clinical features**—The gingiva tissue is typically firm, non-tender, pale pink, and do not bleed easily.
- **Management**—Discontinue medication, if the medication cannot be discontinued, surgical removal of the excess gingiva may be performed but the condition will likely recur.
  Because this condition is worsened by the level of plaque accumulation on the teeth, effective oral hygiene measures should be put in place to reduce the severity.

III. Hereditary gingival fibromatosis:
- **Cause**—Hereditary.

- **Clinical features**—Slow growing generalized or occasionally localized non-tender, firm, pale pink enlargement of the gingiva.
- **Management**—Repeated surgical removal of excess gingiva to avoid impaction and displacement of teeth.

IV. Systemic causes of gingival enlargement:

- **Causes**—Physiological and systemic conditions including pregnancy, hormonal imbalance, and leukaemia (acute myeloid leukaemia).
- **Clinical appearance**—Similar to inflammatory gingiva enlargement.
- **Management**—Treatment of the underlying condition leads to resolution of gingival enlargement. Effective oral hygiene measure if instituted will reduce the risk of developing gingival enlargement.

All the drugs in the option are used to manage hypertension. Amlodipine is a calcium channel blocker, thus the most likely cause of gingival hyperplasia for reasons highlighted earlier. The prevalence of this side effect ranges greatly depending on the type of calcium channel blocker; the risk of which is greatest with nifedipine.

Further reading

The American Academy of Oral Medicine. *Gingival Enlargement*. Available at: https://www.aaom.com/index.php%3Foption=com_content&view=article&id=13 2:gingival-enlargement&catid=22:patient-condition-information&Itemid=120

6. E

NSAIDs, such as ibuprofen, diclofenac, naproxen, and aspirin are cyclooxygenase (COX) inhibitors, with anti-inflammatory and analgesic/antipyretic properties. NSAIDs act reversibly, while aspirin's effects are irreversible. The COX enzyme is responsible for conversion of arachidonic to prostaglandins, which are mediators of pain, inflammation, and fever. Examples of prostaglandins include thromboxane A_2 (which stimulates platelet aggregation and blood clot formation) in platelets and prostacyclin (a vasodilator that inhibits platelet aggregation) in the endothelium, etc.

Two COX isoenzymes (COX-1 and COX-2) are commonly recognized. COX-1 is constitutively expressed and is involved in gastroprotection from stomach acid and in thromboxane formation by platelets. COX-2 is inducible by inflammatory mediators in a wide range of tissues and is constitutively expressed, where it contributes to renal physiology, etc. Blockage of COX-1 and COX-2 effects in tissue where they are constitutively expressed can produce gastric and renal side effects respectively. Hence, non-selective NSAIDs and aspirin are well recognized for their upper gastrointestinal (GI) complications due to loss of the gastroprotective effects conferred by COX-1.

Corticosteroids act by blocking phospholipase A_2 responsible for arachidonic acid production from the phospholipid bilayer. The resultant effect is reduction in the substrate (arachidonic acid) for COX enzymes. Long-term use of corticosteroids also causes increased gastric acid production. The synergistic effects of both drugs when used concurrently, i.e. corticosteroids (increases gastric acid production) with NSAIDs (loss of COX-1 gastric protective effects) can potentially increase the risk of upper gastrointestinal complications (i.e. peptic ulceration and gastrointestinal bleeding).

To mitigate side effect, the dentist must counsel patients on corticosteroids to either avoid or limit the use of NSAIDs (i.e. diclofenac and mefenamic acid in this scenario). Where both medications, must be used concurrently, the general practitioner should consider co-administration of proton pump inhibitors (lansoprazole) for prevention and/or relief of the side effects in at risk patients.

Co-dydramol is not an NSAID but a mixture of two painkiller paracetamol and dihydrocodeine (an opioid). Side effects include constipation, feeling sick, and sleepiness. Most importantly, there is a risk of becoming addicted to the dihydrocodeine in co-dydramol, hence patients using this medication should be regularly reviewed by their doctor.

Considering the untoward effects highlighted earlier, the safest alternative for this patient will be paracetamol, therefore the most plausible option.

Further reading

Scully C. Chapter 7: Gastrointestinal and pancreatic disorders. In: Scully C (ed.). *Scully's Medical Problems in Dentistry*, 7th Edition. Edinburgh, UK: Churchill Livingston/Elsevier, 2014.

7. A

See Table 2.2 for a summary of antihypertensive drugs, their corresponding drug classes, uses, and mechanisms of action.

Table 2.2 Antihypertensive drugs, their corresponding drug classes, uses, and mechanisms of action

Generic name	Drug class	Uses	Mechanisms of action
Ramipril	Angiotensin-converting enzyme inhibitor (ACEI)	Antihypertensive	Reduced generation of angiotensin II (vasoconstrictor) and accumulation of bradykinin (vasodilator). Accumulation of bradykinin Is responsible for dry cough in susceptible individuals
Amlodipine	Calcium channel blocker	Antihypertensive	Acts on vascular smooth muscles resulting in negative inotropy and chronotropy. The resultant effects are peripheral vasodilation and reduced systemic vascular resistance
Gliclazide	Sulfonylurea	Antidiabetic	Augments the secretion of insulin, thus are effective only when there is residual pancreatic beta islet cell activity. It also enhances peripheral insulin sensitivity
Metformin	Biguanide	Antidiabetic	Acts only when there is residual pancreatic beta islet cell activity. It decreases gluconeogenesis in the liver, intestinal absorption of glucose, and increases peripheral utilization of glucose
Simvastatin	Statins	Lipid regulating drug (anticholesterol)	Competitively inhibit 3-hydroxy-3-methylglutaryl coenzyme A (HMG CoA) reductase, an enzyme involved in cholesterol synthesis, especially in the liver

Further reading

BNF Online. Available at: https://www.bnf.org

Jackson RE, Bellamy MC. Antihypertensive drugs. *Cont Educ Anaesthes Crit Care Pain*, 2015;15(6):280–5.

8. B

Lichenoid drug reactions can be associated with many systemic medications, typically, this may occur at any time sometimes up to a year after commencing use of the medication. Some cases have reported to occur after the medication has been stopped making it difficult to identify the culprit medication. See Table 2.3 for examples of medications that can trigger a lichenoid reaction and their corresponding drug classes and uses. Alendronic acid (bisphosphonate drug), co-codamol (analgesic), pioglitazone (antidiabetic drug), simvastatin (lipid-regulating drug) are not typically associated with a lichenoid drug reaction. Therefore, the mostly likely option in this scenario is bendroflumethiazide, a thiazide diuretic used to manage hypertension.

Table 2.3 Examples of medications that can trigger a lichenoid reaction and their corresponding drug classes and uses

Generic names	Drug class	Uses
Ibuprofen, aspirin, indomethacin, naproxen	NSAIDs	Anti-inflammatory, analgesic
Atenolol	Beta blockers	Antihypertensives
Enalapril, ramipril	ACE inhibitors	
Bendroflumethiazide hydrochlorothiazide	Thiazides/diuretics	
Methyl dopa	Centrally acting α_2 adrenoceptor agonist	Management of hypertension in pregnancy
Chlorpropamide Glipizide	Sulfonylureas	Antidiabetics
Metformin	Biguanides	
Allopurinol	Xanthine oxidase enzyme inhibitor	Decrease urate level (management of gout)
Carbamazepine Phenytoin	Anticonvulsants/antiepileptic	Management of epilepsy and neuropathic pain
Gold	Metals/disease-modifying antirheumatic drug (DMARD)	Management of rheumatic arthritis
Hydroxychloroquine Quinine Quinidine	Antimalarials/disease-modifying antirheumatic drug. (DMARD)	Treatment of resistant malaria/management of rheumatic arthritis

Further reading

Scully C. Chapter 29: Materials and drugs. In: Scully C (ed.). *Scully's Medical Problems in Dentistry*, 7th Edition. Edinburgh, UK: Churchill Livingston/Elsevier, 2014.

9. A

Considering all of the medications listed in the options are used for pharmacological management of osteoporosis and related conditions in postmenopausal women, this patient is seeing her rheumatologist for assessment and management of osteoporosis. Some of the medications listed in the options are subject to relatively new regulation limits as discussed in the justifications for the most plausible option, listed next.

Calcitonin is used for long-term treatment of disorders of bone metabolism, such as osteoporosis, Paget's disease, acute bone loss due to sudden immobilization and hypercalcaemia of malignancy. It used to be available as intranasal and injectable formulations. Long-term use of calcitonin in the United Kingdom (UK) has been discontinued because of the absolute increased risk of developing different types of cancer. Calcitonin is still available as a solution for injection and infusion; however, its use is limited to the short-term treatment of:

- Paget's disease—now restricted to patients who do not respond to, or cannot tolerate, alternative treatments (i.e. patients with renal impairment); duration of calcitonin should be limited to up to 3 months, but may be extended to 6 months under exceptional circumstances (e.g. patients with impending pathologic fractures)
- Acute bone loss prevention due to sudden immobilization, for up to 4 weeks only (no change in use)
- Hypercalcaemia of malignancy (no change in use)

Strontium ranelate (Protelos) is used for treatment of severe osteoporosis in postmenopausal women and adult men who are at high risk of fracture. It works by slowing down the breakdown of bone and stimulating the formation of new bone. Similar to alendronic acid, its absorption is affected by food and drink in the stomach, therefore it is advised the medication is taken at least 2 hours after taking food and milk containing drink. In contrast to alendronic acid, there is no need to sit upright after use of the drug. Because of the risk of developing side effects like life-threatening allergic reactions, venous thromboembolism, and increased risk of heart problems, strontium ranelate was discontinued in the UK in August 2017. As at the time of publication of this book, the medication appears to be available for use in the UK again.

Calcium and vitamin D are not used as a sole treatment for patients with osteoporosis, rather they are used as adjunctive treatment for patients who receive treatment with bisphosphonates (alendronate, risedronate), SERMs (raloxifene), strontium ranelate, or teriparatide. The National Institute for Clinical Excellence (NICE) recommends: 'Unless clinicians are confident that women who receive osteoporosis treatment have an adequate calcium intake and are vitamin D replete, calcium, and/or vitamin D supplementation should be provided.'

Hormone replacement therapy can be administered orally and non-orally, no specific precautions are required during oral administration.

Bisphosphonates which includes alendronic acid, zoledronic acid, olpadronate, ibandronic acid, etc. are adsorbed onto hydroxyapatite crystals in bone, slowing both their rate of growth and dissolution, and therefore reducing the rate of bone turnover. The different types are administered via different routes and have specific indications. Alendronic acid is administered via the oral route is used for management of:

- Postmenopausal osteoporosis
- Osteoporosis in men
- Prevention and treatment corticosteroid-induced osteoporosis in postmenopausal women not receiving hormone replacement therapy

In contrast, zoledronic acid is administered by intravenous infusion and used by the specialist only for management of:

- Prevention of skeletal related events in advanced malignancies involving bone
- Tumour-induced hypercalcaemia
- Paget's disease of bone
- Osteoporosis (including corticosteroid-induced osteoporosis) in men and postmenopausal women

Calcitonin and strontium ranelate, while used for management of postmenopausal osteoporosis are both not plausible options. The uses of both medications are currently been discontinued in the UK. Calcium and vitamin D are both used as adjunctive treatment rather than for management of osteoporosis therefore not a plausible option. Oral hormone replacement therapy does not require the precautions in the scenario therefore not plausible. The most plausible option is bisphosphonates specifically alendronic acid, which is administered orally and requires the specific instructions given to this patient. The reasons being food and liquids can reduce its absorption, hence, patients are advised to take the medication with a glass of plain water 30 minutes before the first meal or beverage of the day. To minimize the chances of oesophageal irritation, patients are advised not lie down for at least 30 minutes.

Further reading

Ito A, Yoshimura M. Mechanisms of the analgesic effect of calcitonin on chronic pain by alteration of receptor or channel expression. *Mol Pain*, 2017;13:1744806917720316.

Medicines and Healthcare Products Regulatory Agency. *Calcitonin (Miacalcic): Increased Risk of Cancer with Long-term Use.* Available at: https://www.gov.uk/drug-safety-update/calcitonin-miacalcic-increased-risk-of-cancer-with-long-term-use

Prescribing Advice for GPs. *Strontium Ranelate Discontinued.* Available at: https://www.prescriber.org.uk/2017/06/strontium-ranelate-discontinued/

South-Paul JE, Talabi MB. Chapter 30: Osteoporosis. In: South-Paul JE (ed.). *Current Diagnosis & Treatment in Family Medicine,* 4th Edition. New York, USA: McGraw-Hill Education/Medical, 2015.

10. D

Among all the medications listed (i.e. atorvastatin, lansoprazole, ramipril, aspirin, metformin, and amlodipine) the statins are the drugs to be cautious with when prescribing the antifungal therapy either orally or systemically. The reason being statins (atorvastatin) are metabolized by liver Cytochrome P450, therefore drugs which inhibits this enzyme would increase the serum concentration of statins thereby accentuating their adverse effect. All azole antifungals (miconazole, itraconazole, fluconazole) and macrolide antibiotics (erythromycin, azithromycin, clarithromycin) when used concomitantly with statins increases the risk of rhabdomyolysis (rapid breakdown of skeletal muscle tissue causing elevated levels of creatine kinase) which is pathognomic of statin-induced myopathy. Terbinafine is an antifungal which is used to treat cutaneous candidiasis, dermatophyte infection of the nails, tinea cruris, tinea pedis, etc. It can be applied topically or used orally in tablet form. It is not indicated for treatment of oral candidiasis and there are no known reports of interaction between terbinafine and statins. Therefore, to minimize the risk of this potential drug interaction, a polyene antifungal such as nystatin should be considered as a safe alternative.

Further reading

Dawoud BE, Roberts A, Yates JM. Drug interactions in general dental practice—considerations for the dental practitioner. *Br Dent J,* 2014;216:15–23.

11. D

Although there are the newer novel oral anticoagulants (NOACs) with fewer side effects, drug interactions, and improved safety, warfarin, an oral vitamin K antagonist, is still commonly used by patient's attending general dental practice as:

- Prophylaxis in patients with rheumatic heart disease and atrial fibrillation (AF)
- Prophylaxis after insertion of prosthetic heart valves
- Treatment for venous thrombosis and pulmonary embolism, etc.

Warfarin has important drug interactions that can occur with medications commonly prescribed in the dental practice. They include metronidazole (antimicrobial against anaerobic bacteria and protozoa), macrolide antibiotics (erythromycin, azithromycin, and clarithromycin), amoxicillin and azole antifungals (miconazole, itraconazole, fluconazole). In this patient, the recurrent infection at the angle of the mouth most likely represents oral candidiasis.

All of the medications listed in the options are available for use via the topical route. Betamethasone (corticosteroid), chlorhexidine (antimicrobial), and Difflam (analgesic) are not used for management of oral candidiasis and therefore are not plausible options. Miconazole gel and nystatin are both antifungal drugs, thus can potentially be used to manage this patient recurrent oral candidiasis at the angle of mouth. Nystatin, a polyene antifungal, can be safely prescribed with warfarin and therefore not a plausible option.

Therefore, the most likely culprit for this patient's fluctuating INR is miconazole, an azole antifungal. Azole antifungals inhibit cytochrome P450 required for metabolism of warfarin causing it to remain in its active form for longer together with a decreased clearance. This effect is responsible for the raised, unstable, or oscillating INR readings observed in this patient.

Further reading

National Institute for Health and Care Excellence. *Warfarin.* Available at: https://bnf.nice.org.uk/interaction/warfarin.html

12. B

The enzymes, their tissues of origin, and diagnostic use are shown in Table 2.4.

Table 2.4 List of enzymes, their corresponding tissues of origin, and diagnostic uses

Enzymes	Tissues of origin	Main diagnostic uses
Alanine transferase (ALT)	High levels in the liver, small amounts in the kidney, heart, and muscles	Liver disease (e.g. liver cirrhosis)
Alkaline phosphatase (ALP)	High levels in liver and bone	Liver or bone disease (e.g. liver cirrhosis, Paget's disease) Used in conjunction with other investigations to identify specific ALP isoform, e.g. if other markers of liver disease (ALT, bilirubin, gamma-glutamyl transferase) are raised then the abnormal ALP isoform is most likely of liver origin
Lactate dehydrogenase	Almost all tissues of the body	Cellular injury, not useful for determining cell of origin
Creatinine kinase	Heart, muscle, and brain in three isoforms CK-MB, CK-BB, and CK-MM, respectively	Skeletal muscle damage (e.g. rhabdomyolysis, etc.)
Troponin	Skeletal (troponin C) and heart muscle (troponin T and I)	Cardiac muscle damage (e.g. angina, myocardial infarction)

This patient is on long-term daily medication of simvastatin, aspirin, and bendroflumethiazide for management of hypertension and hypercholesterolaemia. The patient's severe muscular pain is coincident with commencing antibiotic treatment for his spreading dentoalveolar abscess with clarithromycin. Although, the scenario does not specify the reason for the antibiotic choice, it is most likely the patient is allergic to the commonly prescribed penicillin's (amoxicillin).

Clarithromycin, a macrolides antibiotic, is well known and documented for the drug interactions that can arise from concurrent use with simvastatin. It inhibits liver cytochrome P450 and isoenzyme CYP3A4 responsible for metabolizing statins; the resultant effect is an increase exposure to and serum concentration of statins, exacerbating known adverse effect of simvastatin (i.e. myopathy and rhabdomyolysis). Rhabdomyolysis refers to a rapid breakdown of skeletal muscle tissue and release of its cellular constituent, notably creatinine kinase. The result is a significantly raised creatinine kinase level in the blood.

Therefore, the most plausible option is raised creatinine kinase. The other enzymes (lactate dehydrogenase, troponin, alanine transferase, and alkaline phosphatase) are not plausible options as their levels are not known to be impacted by the interaction between clarithromycin and simvastatin. It is imperative that dental practitioners are aware of this serious side effect and consults with the patient's GP for their simvastatin to temporarily be stopped while on clarithromycin or for an alternative antibiotic.

Further reading

Dawoud BE, Roberts A, Yates JM. Drug interactions in general dental practice—considerations for the dental practitioner. *Br Dent J*, 2014;216:15–23.

13. C

Cephalexin is a cephalosporin antibiotic used to treat bacterial infections, including upper respiratory infections, ear infections, skin infections, urinary tract infections, and bone infections. Patients with penicillin allergy are most likely allergic to this drug, therefore this is not a plausible option.

Azithromycin is a broad-spectrum macrolide antibiotic used for the treatment of respiratory, enteric, and genitourinary infections and may be used instead of other macrolides for some sexually transmitted and enteric infections. Azithromycin is structurally related to erythromycin. The only difference being a methyl-substituted nitrogen instead of a carbonyl group at the 9a position on the aglycone ring, which allows for the prevention of its metabolism. This differentiates azithromycin from other types of macrolides (i.e. it does not inhibit cytochrome P450 and is less likely to interact with other drugs).

Erythromycin like azithromycin is a macrolide antibiotic which is used as an alternative in patients with penicillin allergy. Unlike azithromycin, erythromycin inhibits cytochrome p450, a liver enzyme required to metabolize warfarin thereby increasing the anticoagulant effect of warfarin. The BNF describes the severity of interaction as severe and warns practitioners to avoid prescribing. If the medication must be prescribed, practitioners must monitor INR and adjust dose accordingly. In this scenario, erythromycin is the most likely culprit for the patient's raised and fluctuating INR. Other medications prescribed by GDPs that can produce similar effects, i.e. unstable INR and increase risk of bleeding are metronidazole, other macrolide antibiotics (clarithromycin,) and azole antifungals (miconazole, fluconazole).

Trimethoprim is an antibiotic that typically used to treat urinary tract and respiratory tract infections, also used to treat mild to moderate *Pneumocystis jirovecii* (*Pneumocystis carinii*) pneumonia in patients who cannot tolerate co-trimoxazole (in combination with dapsone). According to the BNF, trimethoprim is predicted to increase the anticoagulant effects of warfarin. While this interaction is relevant, trimethoprim is not considered an option as it is less likely to be prescribed for management of dentally related infections.

Vancomycin is a glycopeptide antibiotic with bactericidal activity against aerobic and anaerobic Gram-positive bacteria including multiresistant staphylococci. It is used to treat *Clostridium difficile* infection and as surgical prophylaxis in patients with high risk of methicillin-resistant *Staphylococcus aureus* (MRSA). There are no reported interactions with warfarin and is not likely to be prescribed in a dental setting, and is therefore not a plausible option.

Further reading

National Institute for Health and Care Excellence. *BNF*. Available at: https://bnf.nice.org.uk/

Orofacial manifestations of systemic diseases

14. C

Beckwith–Wiedemann syndrome (BWS) is a congenital overgrowth syndrome that occurs in approximately 1 in 15,000 births. BWS is variable—some children have a number of features of the condition, others have only a few. One of the most common features of the condition is macroglossia (large tongue size). These may cause difficulties with feeding, speech, the development of the teeth and jaws, and increased drooling. Other features which may be associated with this syndrome include higher birth weight, body asymmetry, unusual blood vessels, ear pits, etc.

Cross syndrome is also known as Cross–McKusick–Breen syndrome, depigmentation–gingival fibromatosis–microphthalmia, Kramer syndrome. It is a very rare autosomal recessive genetic trait. It is characterized by hypopigmentation of the skin and hair and abnormalities of the central nervous system that affects the eyes and parts of the brain. Clinical features include light skin colour, silver grey hair, microphthalmia, cornea opacities, and nystagmus. Developmental delays, mental retardation, and spastic paraplegia are also additional features that may develop.

Down's syndrome, also known as trisomy 21, is a genetic disorder caused by the presence of all or part of a third copy of chromosome 21. It is typically associated with physical growth delays, mild to moderate intellectual disability, characteristic facial features, and weak muscle tone (hypotonia) in infancy.

Physical features of Down's syndrome include:

- Eyes that slant upward, have oblique fissures, have epicanthic skin folds on the inner corner, and have white spots on the iris
- Small stature and a short neck
- Single, deep creases across the centre of the palms
- Protruding tongue
- Large space between large and second toe
- Single flexion furrow of the fifth finger
- Congenital heart disease is seen in about 40% of patient with Down's syndrome, most of which are septal defects

Myxoedema is associated with hypothyroidism. Causes of hypothyroidism include autoimmune destruction of the thyroid gland, side effect of treatment for overactive thyroid, thyroid cancer, and less likely congenital hypothyroidism arising abnormal thyroid development or genetic defects in thyroid function. Common signs and symptoms include fatigue, lethargy, cold sensitivity, dry skin and lifeless hair, impaired concentration and memory, increased weight with poor appetite, and constipation. Other features include hoarse voice, tingling of the hands (carpal tunnel syndrome), heavy and late, or absent periods, deafness, and joint aches. These patients can also present a characteristic 'myxoedema facies' in which the face looks puffy due to the accumulation of subcutaneous fluid, cool dry skin, and thinning of the hair including the eyebrows.

Simpson–Golabi–Behmel syndrome is a rare X-linked condition characterized by pre- and postnatal overgrowth, coarse facial appearance, large mouth, predisposition to embryonic neoplasia, and a variety of visceral and skeletal abnormalities. People with Simpson–Golabi–Behmel syndrome have distinctive facial features including widely spaced eyes (ocular hypertelorism), an unusually large mouth (macrostomia), a large tongue (macroglossia) that may have a deep groove or furrow down the middle, a broad nose with an upturned tip, and abnormalities affecting the roof of the mouth (the palate). The facial features are often described as 'coarse' in older children and adults with this condition. Some people with this condition have mild to severe intellectual disability, while others have normal intelligence.

Down's, Beckwith–Wiedemann, and Simpson–Golabi–Behmel syndromes are causes of macroglossia. Myxoedema, if associated with congenital hypothyroidism, can also result in macroglossia. A constellation of all the patient's findings described in the scenario point towards two most likely options, they are both Down's and Simpson–Golabi–Behmel syndromes. However, considering common things are common, the most plausible option for this scenario on the grounds of frequency of occurrence is Down's syndrome.

Further reading

National Organization for Rare Disorders. Available at: https://rarediseases.org

Scully C. Chapter 28: Impairment and disability. In: Scully C (ed.). *Scully's Medical Problems in Dentistry*, 7th Edition. Edinburgh, UK: Churchill Livingston/Elsevier, 2014.

15. E

Gardner syndrome is an inherited as an autosomal-dominant condition. It is characterized by the multiple colorectal polyps which are at risk of transforming into colorectal cancers. Other features include osteomas, epidermoid cysts, lipomas, fibromas, desmoid tumours, adenomatous polyps of the stomach, and adrenal masses. Dental features include multiple impacted and supernumerary teeth, as well as odontomas. Mutation of the *APC* change located in chromosome 5q21 is responsible for this syndrome.

Glanzmann's syndrome also known as Glanzmann disease, Glanzmann–Naegeli syndrome, Glanzmann thrombasthenia is a rare inherited bleeding disorder in which platelets glycoprotein IIB/IIIa, a receptor for fibrinogen is defective or low. The resultant effect is no fibrinogen bridging of platelets to other platelets causing significantly prolonged bleeding time (BT).

Melkersson–Rosenthal syndrome is a rare neurological disorder characterized by a triad of recurrent orofacial swelling (orofacial granulomatosis), relapsing facial paralysis, and fissured tongue. Cheilitis granulomatosa of Miescher is an example of a monosymptomatic variant of the Melkersson–Rosenthal syndrome. The histologic findings of non-caseating, sarcoidal granulomas support the diagnosis.

Peutz–Jeghers syndrome (PJS) is an autosomal-dominant inherited disease characterized by mutation in the *STK11* (*LKB1*) gene. The syndrome is characterized by hamartomatous polyps in gastrointestinal tract which carry a risk of transformation into malignancies. Other features include hyperpigmented macules on the lip and oral mucosa.

Plummer–Vinson (Paterson–Brown–Kelly) syndrome is rare and characterized by the triad of dysphagia, iron deficiency anaemia, and oesophageal webs. Their dysphagia is usually painless, intermittent, or progressive over years, it is limited to solids and can result in weight loss. Symptoms resulting from anaemia include pallor, atrophic glossitis, angular cheilitis, koilonychia, weakness, fatigue, and tachycardia. Patients with Plummer–Vinson syndrome have an increased risk of developing squamous carcinoma of the pharynx and oesophagus. Hence it is imperative these patients are managed with iron supplementation and followed-up closely.

Plummer–Vinson syndrome is the most plausible option as its features closely match those seen in the patient.

Further reading

Scully C. Chapter 8: Haematology. In: Scully C (ed.). *Scully's Medical Problems in Dentistry*, 7th Edition. Edinburgh, UK: Churchill Livingston/Elsevier, 2014.

16. A

Dry skin, thin hair, periorbital puffiness, depression, tiredness, weight gain, muscle ache, being sensitive to cold are clinical features of an underactive thyroid (i.e. hypothyroidism). The most likely oral manifestation in this patient will be macroglossia, this is due to increased accumulation of subcutaneous mucopolysaccharides (i.e. glycosaminoglycans and also due to decrease in their degradation). They can also manifest thickening of lips. Recurrent oral ulcers, median rhomboid glossitis, spaced dentition, and spontaneous gingival bleeding are not clinical features of hypothyroidism, and therefore not plausible options.

Further reading

Wilkinson IB, Wilkinson IB, Raine T, Wiles K, Goodhart A, Hall C, O'Neill H.
Chapter 5: Endocrinology. In: Wilkinson IB, *et al.* (eds). *Oxford Handbook of Clinical Medicine*, 10th Edition. Oxford, UK: Oxford University Press, 2019.

17. C

All the options listed in this scenario have bony involvement. Therefore, the age of the patient, specific imaging, and laboratory findings are important in establishing a definitive diagnosis.

Paget's disease is a chronic localized bone remodelling disorder characterized by increased bone resorption, bone formation, and remodelling, which may lead to major long-bone and skull deformities. It is a disease of the elderly (>50 years). The characteristic radiological appearance is an enlarged bone with coarse trabeculae and thick cortex. Elevated serum alkaline phosphatase is characteristic but not diagnostic.

Langerhans cell histiocytosis (LCH) is a rare disease characterized by the clonal proliferation of pathogenic Langerhans cells and cytokine overproduction. This leads to inflammation and tissue destruction in different organs of the body. The disease can manifest in a single organ system or multiple organs, and commonly involves the bone, skin, lungs, liver, spleen, bone marrow, pituitary gland, and eyes. Typically seen in children but can also affect adults of any age. Radiologically, it can present as a solitary or multiple punched lytic lesion without sclerotic rim. Tissue biopsy with lesional cells highlighted by CD1a S100 and langerin (CD207) is required to establish a definitive diagnosis.

Secondary hyperparathyroidism is a complication of renal failure. It results in hypocalcaemia which in turn triggers the production of parathormone (PTH) and hyperplasia of the parathyroid gland. Bone resorption caused by the increased osteoclast activity and soft tissue calcification are likely manifestations. Brown tumour, with an incidence rate of 0.1%, is also a likely complication. Brown tumour is a giant cell granuloma which appears as a result of the imbalanced osteoclast activity and peritrabecular fibrosis together with hemosiderin deposition into the osteolytic cysts. This lesion rarely involves the craniofacial region but common in the long bones, ribs, and the pelvis. Radiographically the disease can present as solitary or multiple osteolytic lesion (classical 'salt and pepper' appearance and 'ground glass' appearance) as well as decreased density of the bones and a change in normal trabecular pattern. Surgical biopsy is a gold standard in the diagnosis, but radiological findings and biochemical tests (calcium and phosphate levels), including serum PTH, vitamin D level, etc., help in making the diagnosis.

Metastasis to the bone is the third most common site after the lung and liver. Prostate and breast cancer are responsible for most metastatic lesions to the bone. In bone this can present at osteolytic, osteoblastic, and mixed lesions. Osteolytic lesions would be elaborated upon as it is the most relevant to the scenario. Common malignancies associated with osteolytic lesions include multiple myeloma, renal cell carcinoma, lung cancer, non-Hodgkin lymphoma, thyroid cancer, breast cancer, and Langerhans histiocytosis. The bone destruction is mediated by osteoclasts resulting in hypercalcaemia, the most common complication of malignant disease. The mechanisms by which osteolytic lesion develop in malignancies can be via:

- Focal osteolysis by tumour cells
- Generalized osteolysis by humoral factors secreted by the tumour
- Increased renal tubular reabsorption of calcium
- Impaired glomerular filtration

As an example, some breast cancers produce parathyroid hormone-related peptide which can produce osteolytic lesions. Specific lymphoma types can produce active metabolites of vitamin D which increases both bone resorption and intestinal absorption of calcium.

Multiple myeloma (MM) is a plasma cell disorder, characterized by bone marrow infiltration with clonal plasma cells, production of monoclonal immunoglobulin (paraprotein), and end organ damage including lytic lesions in the bones, renal impairment, hypercalcaemia, and anaemia. In MM, lesions could be in the form of a classic discrete lytic lesion (radiolucent, plasmacytoma), widespread osteopenia, or multiple lytic lesions affecting any part of skeleton, preferably spine, skull, and long bones. In the jaw bones, the disease can manifest as root resorption, mental paraesthesia, loosening of teeth. Oral soft tissues swelling including macroglossia, gingiva enlargement have also been reported. This is as a result of deposition of amyloid proteins or infiltration by malignant plasma cells. The identification of Bence-Jones protein in urine and monoclonal IgG in serum using electrophoresis is a distinguishing diagnostic feature.

Therefore, MM is the most plausible option as its features closely match those in the patient described.

Further reading

Macedo F, et al. Bone metastases: an overview. *Oncol Rev*, 2017;11(1):321.

18. C

The constellation of the patient's symptoms and past medical history suggest this patient may have macrocytic specifically megaloblastic anaemia. Megaloblastic anaemia can be caused by impairment or deficiency of vitamin B_{12} or folate.

Vitamin B_{12} deficiency is caused by insufficient dietary intake, malabsorption due to intrinsic factor deficiency caused by pernicious anaemia or following gastric surgery (gastrectomy). Other causes include exposure to nitrous oxide or a congenital disorder such as transcobalamin II deficiency.

Folate deficiency is caused by nutritional deficiency (e.g. poor diet, alcoholism), malabsorption (e.g. coeliac disease, inflammatory bowel disease), increased requirements (e.g. pregnancy, lactation, chronic haemolysis), or medication (e.g. methotrexate, trimethoprim, phenytoin).

Note: The causes of folate deficiency are not linked to previous history of gastric surgery therefore not likely to be a cause of this patient's symptoms.

Also, while both vitamin B_{12} and folic acid deficiency produce similar symptoms (i.e. fatigue, headache, palpitations, dyspnoea, etc.). Neurological symptoms like dysesthesia and hypoaesthesia (peripheral sensory paraesthesia of hands and feet) are generally not seen in folate deficiency. Other symptoms associated with vitamin B_{12} deficiency include Hunter's glossitis and grey hair.

Vitamin B_{12} deficiency requires treatment with parenteral (intramuscular) administration of vitamin B_{12}. For patient with pernicious anaemia or total gastrectomy, lifelong treatment is required. Treatment with oral vitamin B_{12} (hydroxocobalamin) is reported but not yet an established modality.

Oral folic acid for treatment of folate deficiency, oral ferrous fumarate for treatment of iron deficiency anaemia, intramuscular erythropoietin for treatment of patient with anaemia due to chronic kidney disease and blood transfusion to manage patients with severe iron deficiency or acute blood loss.

Therefore, the most plausible option for this scenario is the administration of intramuscular vitamin B_{12}.

Further reading

Hunt A, Harrington D, Robinson S. Vitamin B_{12} deficiency. *BMJ*, 2014;349:g5226.

19. D

All of the conditions listed can present with weight gain, therefore this is not a discriminatory clinical feature.

Patient with severe hypothyroidism may present generalized fatigue and lack of energy (lethargy), muscle weakness and cramping, dryness of the skin and hair, incomplete or infrequent passing of stools (constipation), and sensitivity to cold.

A prolactinoma is a benign tumour of the pituitary gland (adenoma) that produces an excessive amount of the hormone prolactin. In women, they present irregular menstrual periods (oligomenorrhea) or no periods (amenorrhea), infertility, and production of breast milk in women who are not pregnant (galactorrhoea).

Cushing's syndrome is caused by elevated levels of cortisol secondary to an adrenocorticotropic hormone (ACTH)-secreting pituitary tumour (Cushing's disease), autonomous cortisol secretion by the adrenal glands due to adrenocortical neoplasms or hyperplasia, exogenous administration of glucocorticoids, or ectopic ACTH secretion in neoplasia including small cell lung carcinomas and carcinoid tumours. Patient's manifest weight gain around the trunk and face, hump on the back (buffalo hump) due to abnormal deposits of fat, abnormal hair growth (hirsutism), acne, irregular menstruation, increased risk of developing hypertension, type II diabetes mellitus (DM) disease, thinning of skin resulting in stretch marks and easy bruising and neurological problems.

Polycystic ovary syndrome (PCOS) is a heterogeneous disorder seen in premenopausal women characterized a combination of hirsutism (a condition of male-pattern terminal hair growth in women), amenorrhoea (absence of menstruation), chronic anovulation (oligo-anovulation) and infertility, obesity, and enlarged cystic ovaries. The obesity associated with PCOS is due to abdominal adipose tissue deposition and visceral adiposity. This in turn induces insulin resistance and compensatory hyperinsulinism resulting in the development of insulin resistance and type II diabetes. Patient may present obstructive sleep apnoea which causes snoring and daytime fatigue.

Although the condition listed in the options and other aetiologies can present similar clinical features they can be excluded on the following grounds:

Adrenal and ovarian androgen secreting tumours (not in the options) are fortunately rare. Suspicious should arise when symptoms and signs of androgen excess start at any time other than the peripubertal period. Cushing's syndrome can be excluded by clinical judgement. Other options by appropriate biochemical investigations, for example, levels of serum 17-hydroxyprogesterone for non-classic congenital adrenal hyperplasia, prolactin for hyperprolactinaemia, thyroid-stimulating hormone (TSH) for thyroid dysfunction, and follicle-stimulating hormone for premature ovarian failure (hypogonadism).

Therefore, on the grounds of frequency of occurrence (i.e. PCOS is the most plausible option as it is the most common reproductive endocrine disorder of women).

Also, on the basis of the patient's age (i.e. peripubertal to adolescence, the signs and symptoms, e.g. late onset of menstruation, secondary amenorrhoea, and recent onset of sleep apnoea, abnormal hair growth, and use of metformin to manage insulin resistance), the most plausible option also remains polycystic ovary syndrome.

Further reading

Escobar-Morreale HF. Polycystic ovary syndrome: definition, aetiology, diagnosis and treatment. *Nat Rev Endocrinol*, 2018;14(5):270–84.

20. E

Pituitary adenomas can either be microadenomas (<10 mm) or macroadenoma (>10 mm) and giant adenoma (>40 mm). Pituitary adenomas may secrete hormones or cause mass effects. Mass effects include headaches, visual field defects (due to compression on the optic chiasma), and hypopituitarism. Up to two-thirds of pituitary adenomas may secrete hormones including prolactin, growth hormone, adrenocorticotrophic hormone (ACTH). Growth-hormone-producing pituitary adenoma causes acromegaly in more than 95% of patients. The increased secretion of growth hormone stimulates production of insulin-like growth factor (IGF-1) mainly from the liver. Characteristic physical findings in acromegaly include the following: enlargement of hands and feet; change in facial appearance (mandibular prognathism, macroglossia, lip and nose enlargement, forehead prominence, prominent supraorbital ridges); and sweaty and greasy skin. Associated systemic complications include hypertension, cardiomyopathy, DM, carpal tunnel syndrome, arthritis, and sleep apnoea. Gigantism occurs if growth hormone excess begins prior to the closure of the epiphyses during puberty.

Intracranial meningioma and craniopharyngioma are both rare tumours capable of mass effects (i.e. compressing on the pituitary to cause visual defects, however they are less likely to be growth-hormone-producing tumours).

Carcinoid tumours (neuroendocrine carcinoma) and phaeochromocytoma are extrapituitary tumours reported to produce growth hormone releasing hormone (GHRH) causing somatotroph cell hyperstimulation and increased GH secretion. They account for 5% of patient with of acromegaly. However, these patients will present systemic complications of acromegaly (as listed earlier) but not mass effects associated with direct impingement of the pituitary adenomas on adjacent structures like the optic chiasma resulting in visual defects.

Therefore, the most plausible option is pituitary adenoma.

Further reading

Molitch ME. Diagnosis and treatment of pituitary adenomas: a review. *JAMA*, 2017;317(5):516–24.

21. B

Coeliac disease is an autoimmune disease associated with an immune reaction to gluten. The disease primarily affects the small intestine but have broad clinical manifestations which include intestinal and extraintestinal. Classical symptoms include chronic diarrhoea, weight loss, and failure to thrive seen in childhood. Non-classical symptoms iron deficiency, bloating, constipation, chronic fatigue, headache, abdominal pain, and osteoporosis present in childhood or adulthood. A combination of coeliac disease serology testing (IgA-TTG and EMA) and duodenal biopsy (showing increased intraepithelial lymphocytes, crypt hyperplasia, and villous atrophy sampling) is required for the diagnosis of coeliac disease in adults.

Irritable bowel syndrome (IBS) is the most commonly diagnosed gastrointestinal condition. It is a symptom-based condition defined by the presence of abdominal pain or discomfort, with altered bowel habits, in the absence of any other organic disease that cause these sorts of symptoms. Typical features include loose/frequent stools, constipation, bloating, abdominal cramping, discomfort and pain, symptoms brought on by food intake/specific food sensitivities and symptoms dynamic over time (change in pain location, change in stool pattern).

Inflammatory bowel disease (IBD) includes ulcerative colitis and Crohn's disease.

Ulcerative colitis affects the colon and the rectum without involvement of the small intestine and most commonly affects adults aged 30–40. Clinical features include relapsing and remitting mucosal inflammation associated with blood in stool and diarrhoea. Symptoms can include urgency, incontinence, fatigue, increased frequency of bowel movements, mucus discharge, nocturnal defecations, and abdominal discomfort (cramps). Oral manifestations include pyostomatitis vegetans and aphthous-like ulcerations. Establishing a diagnosis of ulcerative colitis is based on a combination of symptoms, endoscopic findings, histology, and the absence of alternative diagnoses. Endoscopy with biopsies is the only way to establish the diagnosis of ulcerative colitis.

Microscopic colitis (MC) is a common cause of chronic, non-bloody diarrhoea which typically affects patients aged 50–60 and occurs more frequently in women than men. The diagnosis is made by both clinical history and endoscopic biopsies. Other common symptom includes abdominal pain, faecal incontinence, and/or weight loss. Colonoscopy generally reveals normal colonic mucosa, but colonic biopsy shows classic histological features: >20 intraepithelial lymphocytes per 100 epithelial cells in lymphocytic colitis and 10–20 μm of a thickened subepithelial collagen band in collagenous colitis.

Crohn's disease is a chronic relapsing remitting condition characterized by transmural inflammation of the intestine and affects any part of the gastrointestinal tract from mouth to perianal area. 25% of the patients have colitis only, 25% is ileitis only and 50% ileocolitis, 33% perianal involvement, and 5–15% with oral or gastroduodenal involvement. It can occur at any age with a peak incidence in the 2–4th decades. Orofacial manifestations include indurated mucosa tag-like lesions, oral ulceration (deep, linear ulceration), glossitis, hyperplasia/thickening of the buccal mucosa and labial fold with a fissuring type appearance ('cobble-stoned' appearance) and diffuse swellings of the lips. Associated clinical symptoms are abdominal pain, fever, diarrhoea, malabsorption, weight loss, and steatorrhea. Extraintestinal manifestations include joint arthritis, uveitis, iritis, episcleritis, erythema nodosum, and pyoderma gangrenosum. The key features for diagnosing Crohn's disease comprises a combination of radiographic, endoscopic, and pathological findings demonstrating focal, asymmetric, transmural, or granulomatous features. Blood investigations will reveal folate or B_{12} deficiency secondary to malabsorption. Raised inflammatory markers such as erythrocyte sedimentation rate (ESR) and C-reactive protein (CRP) used for monitoring the response to treatment and predicting the course of the disease. Faecal granulocyte proteins lactoferrin and calprotectin can also be used to follow-up treatment outcomes.

Note: Faecal calprotectin, a protein detectable in stool that correlates with increased neutrophils in the intestine, can be helpful in ruling out inflammatory bowel disease, However, faecal calprotectin does not distinguish between various causes of intestinal inflammation so cannot be used as a definitive diagnostic tool in Crohn's disease.

Therefore, the most plausible option on the grounds of a constellation of the patient's age, the specific orofacial manifestations, and the presence of raised inflammatory markers and faecal calprotectin (elastase) is Crohn's disease.

Further reading

Gajendran M, Loganathan P, Catinella AP, Hashash JG. A comprehensive review and update on Crohn's disease. *Disease-a-Month*, 2018;64(2):20–57.

Kalla R, et al. Crohn's disease. *BMJ*, 2014;349:g6670.

22. A

Gardner syndrome is an inherited as an autosomal-dominant condition. It is characterized by the multiple colorectal polyps which are at risk of transforming into colorectal cancers. Other features include osteomas, epidermoid cysts, lipomas, fibromas, desmoid tumours, adenomatous polyps of the stomach and adrenal masses. Dental features include multiple impacted and supernumerary teeth as well as odontomas. Others include multiple benign bone osteomas, particularly on the alveolar margin. Mutation of the APC change located in chromosome 5q21 is responsible for this syndrome. Patients born with one mutant APC allele develop thousands of adenomatous polyps in the colon. Somatic mutation of the other allele would result in one or more of the polyps developing colonic cancers. The risk of malignant transformation within the multiple colonic polyps necessities careful follow-up and possible colonic resection/polyp removal.

Gorlin–Goltz syndrome, also known as naevoid basal cell carcinoma syndrome (NBCCS), is an inherited autosomal-dominant condition characterized by lamellar (sheet-like) calcification of the falx, development of multiple jaw keratocysts, frequently beginning in the second decade of life, and/or basal cell carcinomas (BCCs) usually from the third decade onwards. Other features include palmar/plantar pits and a recognizable appearance with macrocephaly, frontal bossing, coarse facial features, and facial milia. Skeletal anomalies (e.g. bifid ribs, wedge-shaped vertebrae), cardiac and ovarian fibromas and medulloblastoma (primitive neuroectodermal tumour), generally the desmoplastic subtype are also characteristic. Identification of a heterozygous germline pathogenic variant in *PTCH1* or *SUFU* on molecular genetic testing establishes the diagnosis if clinical features are inconclusive.

Grinspan syndrome is characterized by the triad essential hypertension, DM, and oral lichen planus. Controversy remains as to whether this is an iatrogenically induced syndrome related to drug therapies for hypertension and DM, both of which are capable on inducing oral lichenoid reactions.

Melkersson–Rosenthal syndrome is a rare neurological disorder characterized by a triad of recurrent orofacial swelling (orofacial granulomatosis), relapsing facial paralysis, and fissured tongue. Cheilitis granulomatosa of Miescher is an example of a monosymptomatic variant of the Melkersson–Rosenthal syndrome. The histologic findings of non-caseating, sarcoidal granulomas support the diagnosis.

PJS is an autosomal-dominant inherited disease characterized by mutation in the *STK11* (*LKB1*) gene. The syndrome is characterized by hamartomatous polyps in gastrointestinal tract as risk of transformation into malignancies. Other features include hyperpigmented macules on the lip and oral mucosa.

The most likely option is therefore Gardener's syndrome.

Further reading

Wilkinson IB, Raine T, Wiles K, Goodhart A, Hall C, O'Neill H. Chapter 15: Eponymous syndromes. In: Wilkinson IB, *et al.* (eds). *Oxford Handbook of Clinical Medicine*, 10th Edition. Oxford, UK: Oxford University Press, 2019.

23. C

All of these syndromes can present characteristic oral and facial features which can facilitate the arrival at a diagnosis. See questions 2 and 9 in the orofacial manifestation of systemic disease section for detailed description of Gardner's, Gorlin–Goltz (naevoid basal cell carcinoma), Peutz–Jeghers, and Plummer–Vinson syndromes.

Albright syndrome (also called McCune–Albright syndrome) affects the skin, bone, and certain endocrine organs. It is characterized by:

- Café-au-lait skin macules which present with jagged and irregular skin pigmentation often referred to as resembling the 'coast of Maine'.
- Fibrous dysplasia which can manifest as monostotic (involvement of one bone) or polyostotic (involvement of more than one bone) disease. This can affect any part and a combination of the craniofacial, axial, and/or appendicular skeleton.
- Endocrine manifestations including precocious puberty, growth hormone excess, neonatal hypercortisolism, thyroid, and testicular lesions.

The diagnosis of Albright syndrome is based on the identification of two or more of the aforementioned clinical features. In individuals whose only clinical finding is monostotic fibrous dysplasia, identification of a somatic activating *GNAS* pathogenic variant is required to confirm the diagnosis.

The most plausible option is Gorlin–Goltz syndrome (NBCCS). These patients develop multiple odontogenic keratocysts in their 20s and develop the first basal cell carcinoma in their 30s.

Further reading

Scully C. Chapter 37: Eponymous and acronymous diseases and signs. In: Scully C (ed.). *Scully's Medical Problems in Dentistry*, 7th Edition. Edinburgh, UK: Churchill Livingston/Elsevier, 2014.

24. C

All of the conditions in the options have either oral or facial manifestations with a bleeding theme.

Angina bullosa haemorrhagia (ABH), a bullous disorder in which recurrent blood blisters of the oropharyngeal mucosa appear in the absence of any identifiable systemic disorder. The lesions occur in adults between 50 and 70 years and typically heal uneventfully within 1 week. The most frequently affected site is the soft palate. Other sites include tongue, buccal and labial mucosa, and floor of mouth. Biopsy from the oral mucosa is usually reported as a subepithelial bulla filled with blood associated with mild to moderate chronic inflammatory infiltrate in the lamina propria. Direct immunofluorescence is always negative. Platelet counts and coagulation tests finding are normal in these patients.

Note: While haemorrhagic blisters can also appear in the setting of leukaemia, vasculitis, and other haematological and haemostatic disorders, ABH is least likely in this scenario.

Bernard–Soulier syndrome (BSS) is a rare inherited platelet bleeding disorder characterized by low platelet count and abnormally large platelets (macrothrombocytopaenia) manifesting as prolonged BT. It is characterized clinically by a history of epistaxis, gingival and cutaneous bleeding, haemorrhage post trauma, and with severe menorrhagia.

PJS is an autosomal-dominant inherited disease characterized by mutation in the *STK11* (*LKB1*) gene. The syndrome is characterized by hamartomatous polyps in gastrointestinal tract as risk of transformation into malignancies. Other features include hyperpigmented macules on the lip and oral mucosa.

Sturge–Weber syndrome (SWS) is also called encephalotrigeminal angiomatosis. It is a neurocutaneous syndrome characterized by angiomas involving the face, choroid, and leptomeninges. The facial capillary vascular malformation is also known as 'port wine stain' or 'nevus flammeus' and usually is seen in the territory of the trigeminal nerve. It is typically unilateral, present at birth, does not change with the age of the patient, and is commonly seen along the ophthalmic or maxillary segment of the trigeminal nerve (forehead, cheeks). Seizures in the first year of life and glaucoma are also characteristic findings. SWS is caused by a somatic mutation in GNAQ.

Hereditary haemorrhagic telangiectasia (HHT) (also known as Osler–Weber–Rendu syndrome) is an autosomal-dominant disorder characterized by multiple mucocutaneous telangiectasias (dilated blood vessels that appear as thin spiderweb-like red and dark purple lesions that blanch with pressure). Telangiectasias appear after puberty and typically occur on the face, lips, tongue, palms, and fingers. They represent small arteriovenous malformations (abnormal connections between arteries and veins that bypass the capillary system) that frequently tend to bleed. Patients typically present with nose bleeds, gastrointestinal bleeds, and iron-deficiency anaemia.

Bernard–Soulier syndrome and Osler–Weber–Rendu syndrome are both likely options on the grounds of experiencing bleeding episodes like epistaxis and menorrhagia. However, the multiple telangiectatic spots are characteristic of the latter syndrome. The absence of low platelet counts and abnormally large platelets (macrothrombocytopaenia) in the patient's full blood count and peripheral smear excludes Bernard–Soulier syndrome. Therefore, the most plausible option is Osler–Weber–Rendu syndrome (HHT).

Further reading

Scully C. Chapter 37: Eponymous and acronymous diseases and signs. In: Scully C (ed.). *Scully's Medical Problems in Dentistry*, 7th Edition. Edinburgh, UK: Churchill Livingston/Elsevier, 2014.

25. E

See questions 2 and 9 of the orofacial manifestation of systemic disease section for detailed description of Gardner's and Melkersson–Rosenthal syndrome.

PJS is an autosomal-dominant disorder characterized by hamartomatous gastrointestinal polyposis and melanin pigmentation of the skin and mucous membranes. The polyps occur throughout the whole digestive tract with a predilection for the small bowel but have also been found in urinary tract, uterus, biliary tract, and nasal mucosa. These polyps can rapidly increase in size to cause recurrent intussusceptions or intestinal obstruction and most patients present in adolescence or young adulthood with episodes of colicky abdominal pain.

Pigmentation of skin and mucous membranes is the external hallmark of PJS. Irregularly distributed light to dark brownish macules of 1–5 mm diameter occurs most commonly on the lips and oral mucosa (mainly the buccal mucosa, gums, and hard palate), but smaller and darker macules can also be found around the mouth, nose, and eyes. Slightly larger pigmented macules can occur on the palms and soles, volar aspects of the fingers and toes, and occasionally on the external genitalia. Mucocutaneous pigmentation starts to appear in infancy or early childhood, reaching a maximum at puberty. The oral lesions usually persist whereas the pigmentation on the skin and lips typically tends to fade. Biopsy of the pigmented skin macules shows an increase in basal layer keratinocyte pigmentation but no increase in melanocyte number.

There is a significantly increased risk of malignancy, at both gastrointestinal as well as extraintestinal sites. Gastrointestinal sites commonly affected are the large bowel, duodenum, and stomach whereas extraintestinal cancer sites include the breasts, uterus, cervix, ovaries, testicles, and pancreas. To ensure polyps are identified early and removed, comprehensive screening protocols consisting of two yearly upper and lower gastrointestinal endoscopy and small bowel follow through, early breast screening, and yearly gynaecological evaluation is recommended. Germline mutations in the serine threonine kinase *STK11* (previously denoted as *LKB1*) located on chromosome 19p13.3 is associated with PJS.

Laugier–Hunziker syndrome is a sporadic condition characterized by acquired and benign melanotic pigmentation of the oral cavity and lips together with spotted macular pigmentation of the fingertips and longitudinal melanonychia. The syndrome is acquired and appears in early to mid-adult life and there is no association with systemic disease. Biopsy of lesions shows increased melanin deposition in basal layer keratinocytes and dermal pigmentary incontinence as well as an increase in the number of melanophages in the papillary dermis, but no increase in the number of melanocytes.

Addison's disease (AD) also known as primary adrenal insufficiency is a chronic disorder of the adrenal cortex resulting in inadequate secretion of glucocorticoid and mineralocorticoid. In the developed world, it is mostly associated with autoimmune disease, while in developing countries tuberculosis is the most common aetiology. Clinical symptoms include weight loss, anorexia, fatigue, diarrhoea, nausea, vomiting, and abdominal pain, etc. Signs include skin and mucosa pigmentation, weight loss, postural hypotension, vitiligo.

Intestinal polyps are associated with Gardner and PJSs, however the former is not associated with pigmentation of skin and mucous membranes. Laugier–Hunziker syndrome is associated with pigmentation of skin and mucous membranes similar to PJS but is not associated with systemic disease, intestinal polyposis, and more specifically the germline mutation of *STK11* (*LKB1*) gene characteristic seen in PJS. Melkersson–Rosenthal syndrome is not associated with any of the features described in this patient, and is therefore not considered an option. AD is also not an option as the patient is asymptomatic and also intestinal polyps are not a feature. Therefore, the most plausible option for this patient is PJS as they exhibit pigmentation of skin and mucous membranes together with hamartomatous gastrointestinal polyposis, which warrants regular gastrointestinal endoscopic screening with a view to performing prophylactic polypectomy.

Further reading

Lampe AK, Hampton PJ, Woodford Richens K, Tomlinson I, Lawrence CM, Douglas FS. Laugier–Hunziker syndrome: an important differential diagnosis for Peutz Jeghers syndrome. *J Med Genet*, 2003;40(6):e77.

Wilkinson IB, Raine T, Wiles K, Goodhart A, Hall C, O'Neill H. Chapter 15: Eponymous syndromes. In: Wilkinson IB, *et al.* (eds). *Oxford Handbook of Clinical Medicine*, 10th Edition. Oxford, UK: Oxford University Press, 2019.

26. C

Addison's disease, also known as primary adrenal insufficiency, is a chronic disorder of the adrenal cortex resulting in inadequate secretion of glucocorticoid and mineralocorticoid. Patients with AD present skin and mucosa pigmentation alongside other features described in question 12 of the orofacial manifestation of systemic disease section. It is not a childhood disease and does not present multiple skin nodules, and therefore not considered plausible option.

Basal cell carcinoma may present as multiple skin lesions in syndromic patients (i.e. Gardener syndrome), but do not present skin and mucosal pigmentation and is also not a childhood disease. See questions 2 and 9 from the orofacial manifestation of systemic disease section for a detailed description of Gardner syndrome.

PJS is a hereditary syndrome associated with pigmentation of the skin and mucous membranes. Although lesions appear in infancy or early childhood, they are macular (flat) lesions and not associated with multiple skin nodules. (See question 12 of the orofacial manifestation of systemic disease section for detailed description of PJS.)

Neurofibromatosis is a heterogeneous group of hereditary cancer syndromes that lead to tumours of the central and peripheral nervous systems. There are three subtypes: neurofibromatosis type 1 (NF1, 96%), neurofibromatosis type 2 (NF2, 3%), and a lesser known form, schwannomatosis.

Neurofibromatosis type 1, also known as Von Recklinghausen disease or peripheral neurofibromatosis, is an autosomal-dominant condition characterized by the development of multiple neurofibromas of the peripheral nerves (varying size dome-shaped violaceous nodules). Other features include café-au-lait macules, freckling in the axillary and inguinal areas, Lisch nodules (iris hamartomas), optic glioma, and a distinctive osseous lesion. Patients with two or more of these features, including having a first relative with NF1, are diagnosed clinically with NF1. NF1 is caused by a mutation in the neurofibromin tumour suppressor gene located on chromosome 17.

Café-au-lait spots are benign tan brown macules which can occur anywhere on the body; most patients with NF1 would present six or more of these in childhood. The neurofibroma in NF1 may be cutaneous or internal (i.e. involving deep tissues like gastrointestinal tract, retroperitoneum, mediastinum, etc.). Plexiform neurofibromas often develops in childhood and are pathognomic of NF1. This type of neurofibroma rather than growing intraneurally within a single nerve, grows to involve multiple fascicles or branches of a nerve or plexus. They grow rapidly and can exert mass effects (compression), they also carry an increased risk of malignant transformation to malignant peripheral nerve sheath tumour (MPNST).

NF2, also known bilateral acoustic neurofibromatosis or central neurofibromatosis, is a hereditary tumour syndrome characterized predominantly by the development of schwannomas, along with meningiomas, ependymomas, and ocular abnormalities. Despite the name, neurofibromas are relatively infrequent. NF2 is inherited in an autosomal-dominant pattern. Patients usually present around age 20. The disease is caused by a mutation in the *NF2* gene on chromosome 22, which encodes for a protein, merlin. Bilateral schwannomas of the superior vestibular branch of the eighth cranial nerve (vestibular schwannoma or acoustic neuroma) are pathognomonic for NF2.

Schwannomatosis is a syndrome characterized by the development of multiple peripheral nerve schwannomas, without concomitant involvement of the vestibular nerve. It is caused by a germline mutation in the *SMARCB1* gene located on chromosome 22q11.2.

Tuberous sclerosis complex (TSC) is a complex childhood and genetically determined disorder characterized by the formation of hamartomas in multiple organs. The most common organs involved are the brain, skin, kidneys, retina, and heart. TSC exhibits autosomal-dominant inheritance and is caused by mutation in either chromosomes 9q34 (TSC1) and 16p13 (TSC2) leading to dysfunction of hamartin or tuberin, respectively. Hamartin and tuberin form a protein complex that helps to regulate cellular hyperplasia.

- Neurological manifestations: Epileptic seizures, neurological tubers
- Renal manifestations: Angiomyolipoma, polycystic kidney disease
- Cardiac manifestations: Cardiac rhabdomyomas
- Pulmonary manifestations: Lymphangioleiomyomatosis
- Dermatological manifestations: Hypomelanotic macules, angiofibroma's, shagreen patches, forehead plaques, and ungual fibromas
- Ophthalmological manifestations: Retinal astrocytic hamartoma
- Miscellaneous: Oral fibroma

To summarize, basal cell carcinoma does not present in childhood and is not associated pigmented spots and multiple nodules, so not a plausible option. AD although associated with skin and mucosal pigmentation is not a childhood disease and not characterized by multiple skin nodules. Patients with Addison's can also present typical clinical features such as nausea, vomiting, abdominal pain, hypotension, hypoglycaemia, etc., thus can be excluded. PJS is associated with macular pigmentation of the skin and mucous membranes which can develop in childhood but do not exhibit multiple nodular skin lesions, therefore not a plausible option. Tuberous sclerosis and neurofibromatosis are both genetically determined disorders with an autosomal-dominant inheritance pattern which manifest as hamartomatous growth and pigmented lesions involving the skin. That said, tuberous sclerosis presents hypomelanocytic skin macules. Therefore, the most plausible option on the basis of pigmentation of skin lesions (café-au-lait spots) and painless skin nodules (neurofibroma) which increase with age is neurofibromatosis.

Further reading

Wilkinson IB, Raine T, Wiles K, Goodhart A, Hall C, O'Neill H. Chapter 10: Neurology. In: Wilkinson IB, *et al.* (eds). *Oxford Handbook of Clinical Medicine*, 10th Edition. Oxford, UK: Oxford University Press, 2019.

27. B

Down's syndrome (DS) is a chromosome disorder associated with an extra chromosome (Trisomy 21) resulting in intellectual disability and specific physical features. DS is one of the most common genetic abnormalities, affecting approximately 1 in 700–800 live births.

Oral manifestations:

- Early onset severe periodontal disease
- Delayed eruption of permanent teeth
- Malocclusion
- Congenitally missing and malformed teeth are common
- Hypoplasia of mid-facial region
- Hypodontia, microdontia
- Macroglossia, fissured and protruding tongue
- Tongue thrust, bruxism, clenching, mouth breathing
- Severe malocclusion (Class III malocclusion)

Facial manifestations:

- Flatten facial profile and nose
- Small head, ear, and mouth
- Upward slanting eyes, often with a skin fold that comes out from the upper eyelid and covers the inner corner of the eye
- White spots on the coloured part of the eye (called Brushfield spots)

Ectodermal dysplasia is used to designate a heterogenous group of disorders characterized by a constellation of findings involving a primary defect of the skin, teeth, and appendageal structures including hair, nail, exocrine, and sebaceous glands. Ectodermal dysplasia is transmitted as a sex-linked recessive trait with females being gene carriers and disease manifestation in males. Characteristic features include hypohidrosis resulting in heat intolerance and occasional hyperpyrexia; smooth, soft, dry, and thin skin; fine, blond, short, and stiff hair over the scalp. They have increased susceptibility to allergic disorders like asthma or eczema. Facial manifestations include frontal bossing, depression of nasal bridge, protuberant lips, and obliquely placed ears, missing eyelashes and eyebrow hairs. Oral manifestations are oligodontia which is the most striking feature. Anodontia is reported but extremely rare. Conical shaped teeth with thin enamel are present.

Ehlers–Danlos syndrome is a heritable connective tissue disorder which is inherited in autosomal-dominant pattern. Typical features include skin hyperextensibility, joint hypermobility (i.e. dislocations and subluxations), easy bruising or bleeding, poor wound healing manifesting as skin rhytids and aberrant scarring, gastrointestinal issues like hiatal hernia or prolapse. Patients with a specific subtype can present characteristic facies which include prominent eyes, lobeless ears, and widened nasal bridge.

Fibrous dysplasia is a benign intramedullary fibro-osseous lesion. It is a bone developmental anomaly characterized by replacement of normal bone and marrow by fibrous tissue. It can involve any of the bones as a single lesion (monostotic) or in multiple bone lesions (polyostotic) or all of the skeletal system (panostotic) and the craniofacial form. In the craniofacial region, the zygomatic-maxillary complex is the most commonly involved. Fibrous dysplasia is not heritable but caused by post-zygotic mutation in the GNAS1 gene. Clinical manifestations include facial asymmetry due to deformity of craniofacial bone, as abnormal bone growth can cause encroachment on cranial nerves. Features will depend on what nerve is compressed. Typical features can include vision changes, hearing impairment, pain, paraesthesia, nasal congestion, and or obstruction. Fibrous dysplasia may be associated with McCune–Albright syndrome where they present extraskeletal manifestations including café-au-lait spots and endocrinopathies.

Pierre Robin syndrome is characterized by micrognathia (mandibular hypotrophy), glossoptosis (abnormal posterior placement of the tongue), obstruction of the upper airways, and cleft palate. Pierre Robin syndrome is not associated with any single underlying pathogenesis or gene mutation; rather, it is a disorder where multiple malformations results from a sequential chain of malformation. In this case, micrognathia leads to glossoptosis which in turn results in airway obstruction, inability to feed, and a U-shaped cleft palate. These craniofacial anomalies can occur in association with other syndrome including Treacher Collins, velocardiofacial, and Stickler syndromes.

While hypodontia can be a feature in both DS and ectodermal dysplasia, scant fine hair, absence of eyelashes and eyebrows, and dry skin are characteristic features of ectodermal dysplasia. Therefore, ectodermal dysplasia is the most plausible option.

Further reading

Scully C. Chapter 11: Mucosal, oral and cutaneous disorders. In: Scully C (ed.). *Scully's Medical Problems in Dentistry*, 7th Edition. Edinburgh, UK: Churchill Livingston/Elsevier, 2014.

28. E

An epulis refers to a localized gingival swelling. There are various types which cannot be distinguished clinically with certainty, hence histological evaluation is required to establish their true nature.

Fibrous epulis also known as irritation fibroma or fibroepithelial polyps usually result from local gingival irritation, leading to fibrous hyperplasia. They are typically pink and firm.

Pyogenic granulomas are usually softer and redder and represent a vascularized reaction to local factors including inadequate oral hygiene, malocclusion, orthodontic appliances, and in pregnancy. During pregnancy, gingivitis can worsen or even result in a pyogenic granuloma which is a harmless overgrowth of large numbers of tiny blood vessels. Typically, the lesions are partially ulcerated, bright red, have a bumpy surface, and have the propensity to ooze and bleed when accidentally traumatized. They tend to appear in the second month and resolve post parturition. Where the lesion persists post pregnancy, it needs to be excised. *Note*: fibrous and pregnancy epulis are not synonymous lesions

Giant cell granulomas also known as giant cell tumours are reactive lesions typically seen in children and caused by local irritation. Histologically, the lesion is characterized by proliferation of giant cells in a background of inflamed fibrous tissue. Clinically, it has a deeper red colour and tends to arise interdentally especially in the premolar region.

Gingiva hypertrophy may represent a localized (malocclusion, inadequate oral hygiene) or generalized process (hereditary condition like gingival fibromatosis), or be secondary to medications like the use of calcium channel blockers (i.e. nifedipine), or anticonvulsants (phenytoin).

Pregnancy gingivitis is usually an exaggerated inflammatory response to local irritation factors in response to a surge in oestrogen and progesterone during pregnancy. Similar lesions can be seen at puberty, in patients on oral contraceptive pills, and those on hormone replacement therapy. This typically present as red and swollen gums which bleed on slight provocation like tooth brushing.

This lesion may worsen to become a pyogenic granuloma, however until this happens it is not a gingival lump, therefore not a plausible option.

Pyogenic granuloma is the most plausible option on clinical grounds (i.e. localized gingival lump, associated with pregnancy, and tendency towards bleeding). However, an excisional biopsy for histological assessment may be required if the lesion persists after parturition.

Further reading

Scully C. *Oral and Maxillofacial Medicine-E-Book: The Basis of Diagnosis and Treatment.* London, UK: Elsevier Health Sciences, 2012.

Haematological diseases

29. C

The patient's clinical features match those seen in infectious mononucleosis. Infectious mononucleosis also known as kissing disease or glandular fever is caused by Epstein–Barr virus (EBV) and typically seen in older children and young adult. The infection can be spread by coming in contact with infected saliva through kissing. Splenomegaly evident on ultrasonography if not on palpation, occurs in almost all cases of infectious mononucleosis, and the risk of splenic rupture is well established. In the scenario, abdominal pain in a setting of infectious mononucleosis and investigation findings of splenomegaly establishes this patient is at risk of potentially serious and lethal complication like a spontaneous rupture or atraumatic rupture of the spleen. Therefore, timely surgical intervention to remove the spleen can prevent potential patient death. In cases, where splenomegaly is not evident, patient who are typically young (15–21 years old) are advised to avoid strenuous or contact sports (swimming, football, rugby, diving) or activities associated with increased intra-abdominal pressure such as weightlifting for up to 8 weeks. It is prudent to mention here that the incidence of splenic rupture is less than 1% and most tend to occur in the initial three weeks of the infection. Other indications for a splenectomy include trauma, splenic abscess, splenic cyst, Hodgkin's disease, chronic myeloid leukaemia, chronic lymphocytic leukaemia, haemoglobinopathies like sickle cell disease, thalassemia, erythrocyte membrane disorders like hereditary spherocytosis, thrombocytopenic purpura, Felty's syndrome, autoimmune thrombocytopenia, etc. However, these indications are unlikely to present in combination with the other features described in this patient. Therefore, the most plausible option is infectious mononucleosis.

Further reading

Lennon P, Crotty M, Fenton JE. Infectious mononucleosis. *BMJ*, 2015;350:h1825.

30. B

Warfarin is a vitamin K antagonist used to achieve anticoagulation in patient with AF. Its anticoagulant effect is monitored by measuring INR. In this scenario, the patient warfarin is outside the therapeutic range because they have accidentally taken too much. Other potential causes for a high patient's INR include:

- Drug interactions with other medicines (e.g. miconazole gel, antibiotics, steroids)
- Concomitant use of alcohol
- Concomitant use of herbal remedies (St. John's wort, glucosamine, chloral, etc.)
- Food or drink intake (cranberry juice, green vegetables, etc.)
- General health (e.g. weight loss, gastroenteritis, smoking cessation all of which can increase the effect of warfarin)

NICE guidelines for management of the patient with high INR reading as in this scenario are as summarized next:

INR >8.0 with the absence of or minor bleeding

- Discontinue warfarin
- Administer 0.5–1 mg vitamin K by slow IV injection or 5 mg by mouth
- Repeat vitamin K injection after 24 hr if INR is still high
- Resume warfarin when the INR <5.0

INR 6.0–8.0 or <6.0 but >0.5 units above the target value:

- Discontinue warfarin
- Resume warfarin when the INR <5.0

Therefore, the most plausible option on the basis of the NICE recommendations is to stop warfarin and administer oral vitamin K.

Further reading

National Institute for Health and Care Excellence (NICE). Anticoagulation—oral. Scenario: warfarin. Available at: http://cks.nice.org.uk/anticoagulation-oral#!scenario:4

31. E

BT is used to assess platelet function.

Full blood count is a measure of the numbers of cells in blood, including RBCs, white blood cells, and platelets.

Clotting factor assays is used to assess for specific coagulation factor deficiency.

Activated partial thromboplastin time (APTT) is a measure of the functionality of the intrinsic and common pathways of the coagulation cascade.

Prothrombin time (PT) may also be called INR test, INR stands for a way of standardizing the results of PT tests, no matter the testing method. It permits interpretation of results in the same way even when they come from different laboratories and different test methods. PT/INR is used to assess factors I, II, V, VII, and X, or the extrinsic coagulation cascade.

Prothrombin, factor II is produced in the liver and is a vitamin K dependent clotting factor like factors I, V, VII, and X. Warfarin is a vitamin K antagonist, therefore patient on this medication will present a high PT/INR.

Despite this patient's polypharmacy, warfarin stands out as the most likely to cause post-extraction bleeding. Warfarin action is assessed by measuring INR which can be checked on the day of operation or if not possible, within 24–72 hours prior to the surgical procedure. This can be done at the chair-side using the CoaguChek XS system self-testing device. The normal INR is 1 and any levels above this indicates clotting will take longer. The normal therapeutic INR for AF patients on warfarin is 2–3. Levels >4 is non-therapeutic and requires adjustment of the warfarin dose by the patient's general medical practitioner or haematologist. Furthermore, UK Medicines Information (UKMI) recommends patients with INR >4 should not have a dental procedure in primary care.

Therefore, the most likely test requested for this patient before proceeding with an extraction is PT which also refers to the INR.

Further reading

Meechan JG, Greenwood M. General medicine and surgery for dental practitioners' part 9: haematology and patients with bleeding problems. *Br Dent J*, 2003;195(6):309.

32. A

Haemophilia A and B are both sex-linked bleeding disorders associated with factor VIII and IX deficiency due to mutations in the F8 and F9 genes, respectively. It is rare and affects 1 in 10,000 births worldwide. Residual factor level correlates directly with bleeding phenotype wherein patients with severe disease (<1%) present with spontaneous bleeds as is the case with this patient; those with moderate disease (1–5%) bleed with minor trauma and rarely spontaneously; and those with mild disease (6–30%) bleed only secondary to trauma or invasive procedures. See question 3 of the haematological diseases section for details of bleeding investigations and what they are used to assess. Factor VIII and IX are part of the intrinsic pathway; therefore, haemophiliac patients are mostly likely to have a prolonged APTT. The INR will be normal as the extrinsic pathway which is used to assess vitamin K dependent factors (I, II, V, VII X) is not affected; also the BT and Von Willebrand factor are normal as platelets count and function are within normal limits in haemophilia.

Further reading

Fijnvandraat K, Cnossen MH, Leebeek FW, Peters M. Diagnosis and management of haemophilia. *BMJ*, 2012;344:e2707.

33. E

Table 2.5 List of the patient's medications in question 5, their corresponding classes, and uses

Drugs	Classes	Uses
Atenolol	β adrenergic block	Antihypertensive
Amlodipine	Calcium channel blocker	Antihypertensive
Simvastatin	Statin	Lowering blood cholesterol
Aspirin	Acetyl salicylic acid	Analgesic/antipyretic—high doses Antiplatelet (blood thinning)—low dose as prophylaxis for patient at high risk of heart attack and strokes

As a general rule it is always prudent to consult with the patient's general medical practitioner before requesting a patient stops any medication prior to having dental treatment. In this patient, the requirement of an emergency extraction prevents prior consultation and stoppage of any medication's days before the treatment. Based on the classes and use of the patient's medication as shown in Table 2.5, prophylactic aspirin at low dose is the most likely to impact on the emergency extraction because of its antiplatelet (blood thinning) properties.

Aspirin induces a permanent functional defect in platelets detected clinically as prolonged BT. This irreversible effect of aspirin on platelets may take up to 10 days to clear from the system as the average lifespan of a platelet is about 8–10 days.

The effects of aspirin vary with the dose, at low doses, 75 mg, cyclooxygenase (COX-1) is blocked thereby inhibiting platelet generation of thromboxane A2, resulting in an antithrombotic effect. At higher doses both COX-1 and COX-2 are inhibited thereby blocking prostaglandins production and producing analgesic and antipyretic effects.

Aspirin affects primary haemostasis only (i.e. the formation of the initial platelet plug), and therefore prolongs BT only. It has no impact on the INR used to assess the extrinsic coagulation cascade. Aspirin in low doses (75 mg) used as a prophylactic measure by patients with cardiovascular disease does not normally need to be stopped prior to an extraction, this is because the risk of thrombosis far outweighs the bleeding associated with dentistry. Hence there is no need to consult the patient's GP via telephone before the extraction. In this patient the use of local measures such as suturing and packing with a haemostatic agent is recommended to prevent post-extraction haemorrhage. The provision of clear oral and written instructions as to what to do in the event of a bleeding episode post extraction is a requisite and of utmost importance.

Further reading

Meechan JG, Greenwood M. General medicine and surgery for dental practitioners' part 9: haematology and patients with bleeding problems. *Br Dent J*, 2003;195(6):309.

34. C

The parameters in the patient's full blood count results which are abnormal are, the mean cell volume (MCV), 125 fl (80–100 fl) and the peripheral blood smear showing megaloblasts and hypersegmented neutrophils. Both are characteristic of megaloblastic anaemia. Megaloblastic anaemia without neuropathy is classically associated with folate deficiency. In this homeless alcoholic patient who has lived rough for about a year, their folate deficiency is probably due to a combination of factors including reduced dietary intake, intestinal malabsorption, reduced liver uptake and storage, and increased urinary excretion. Folate deficiency facilitates progression of alcoholic liver disease by reducing antioxidant defences as well as contributing to DNA instability through abnormalities in methionine metabolism and the methylation regulation of relevant gene expressions. Therefore, a liver function test to assess for alcoholic liver disease and folate levels to confirm the deficiency state most likely to be causative of the patient's oral manifestations (i.e. recurrent oral ulcerations and angular cheilitis is prudent).

Ferritin and iron studies are used to assess for microcytic anaemia. Urea and electrolytes, magnesium, and zinc are most likely to be within normal range. Although serum B_{12} deficiency can present similar oral manifestations described in this patient, it is unlikely to be abnormal for two reasons:

- Patient has no neuropathic manifestations
- Serum B_{12} body stores can last around 2–4 years without being replenished, hence the manifestations of deficiency can take a longer time (i.e. >1 year since this patient started sleeping rough).

Therefore, the most plausible option is liver function test and serum folate.

Further reading

BMJ Best Practice. Folate deficiency. Available at: https://bestpractice.bmj.com/topics/en-gb/823

Medici V, Halsted CH. Folate, alcohol, and liver disease. *Mol Nutr Food Res*, 2013;57(4):596–606.

35. C

The patient's oral manifestations are suggestive of a nutritional deficiency. Folate and vitamin B_{12} deficiency present similar clinical features with the exception of neurological symptoms. The patient's lip paraesthesia is a neurological manifestation likely to be related to vitamin B_{12} deficiency.

Cause of vitamin B_{12} deficiency and their corresponding pathogenesis include:

- Pernicious anaemia: insufficient B_{12} absorption caused by a deficiency of intrinsic factor due to autoimmune destruction of gastric parietal cells.
- Gastric disease or surgery (partial or complete gastrectomy or gastric reduction surgery): insufficient B_{12} absorption caused by a diminished production of intrinsic factor due to decreased number of gastric parietal cells.
- Chronic atrophic gastritis (chronic inflammation causing loss of the gastric acid-producing cells) and an intake of drugs that affect gastric acid secretion or gastric pH (that is, proton pump inhibitors, histamine receptor 2 antagonists and antacids): Vitamin B_{12} is not released from the food matrix owing to insufficient hydrochloric acid and low pepsin activity.
- Pancreatic disease or pancreatectomy: Vitamin B_{12} is not released from the haptocorrin complex owing to insufficient pancreatic enzyme activity.
- Other intestinal diseases, ileal resection, parasitic infestations, and bacterial overgrowth: impaired absorption of the vitamin B_{12}–intrinsic factor complex.
- Medications that affect vitamin B_{12} absorption or metabolism: reduction of serum vitamin B_{12} levels via known mechanisms (for example, cholestyramine) and unknown mechanisms (for example, metformin).

- Dietary factors such as general malnutrition, vegetarian or vegan diet, and chronic alcoholism: reduced vitamin B_{12} consumption.
- Inherited disorders: decreased expression, binding activity, or affinity of receptors and proteins involved in vitamin B_{12} trafficking and metabolism
- Miscellaneous: including HIV infection and nitrous oxide anaesthesia.

Intrinsic factor (IF) secreted by gastric parietal cells binds to vitamin B_{12}, the complex formed is absorbed in the terminal ileum. Therefore, a complete ileectomy as treatment for the patient's Crohn's disease would impair B_{12} absorption resulting in the patient's oral manifestations. Therefore, the most plausible option for this patient's deficiency state and oral manifestation is malabsorption.

Further reading

Green R, et al. Vitamin B 12 deficiency. *Nat Rev Dis Primers*, 2017;3:17040.

36. E

Sickle cell anaemia exhibits an autosomal recessive mode of inheritance and is caused by a mutation in chromosome 11 that results in the replacement of glutamic acid with valine at position 6 of the N-terminus of the globin chain. The manifestations of sickle cell anaemia are:

- Painful vaso-occlusive crises caused by obstruction of the microvasculature by sickled RBCs, causing ischaemia and pain.
- Microinfarcts caused by sickling most commonly affect the spleen, kidney, skeleton, and central nervous system. Obstruction of the microvasculature in the spleen renders patients functionally asplenic and susceptible to infection, particularly with encapsulated bacteria such as *Streptococcus pneumonia*, *Escherichia coli*, *Haemophilus*, and *Meningococcus*.
- Haemolytic anaemia caused by chronic intravascular haemolysis resulting in a reduced lifespan of the abnormal RBCs (10–20 days compared with 100–120 days in a healthy adult). It may be complicated by megaloblastic changes caused by folate deficiency.
- End organ damage caused by vasculopathy and tissue ischaemia.

In this patient:

- Bone pain is as a result of a vaso-occlusive crisis and not a bone infection (alveolar osteitis).
- Jaundice is a consequence of massive RBC haemolysis manifesting as increased unconjugated bilirubin in serum seeping into tissue and not glucose-6-phosphate dehydrogenase deficiency.
- Glossitis is a manifestation of anaemia arising from iron and folate deficiencies and not vitamin B_{12} deficiency.
- Gallstones is a consequence of chronic RBC haemolysis which leads to continuous production of bilirubin, which is conjugated in the liver and excreted in the faeces as urobilinogen; in large quantities, it may form calcium bilirubinate gallstones.
- Maxillary prognathism is a consequence of compensatory extramedullary haematopoiesis aimed at increasing erythroid production to correct for the rapid loss of RBCs via intravascular haemolysis.

Therefore, maxillary prognathism and erythroid hyperplasia is the most plausible option as both the clinical feature and corresponding pathophysiology best match.

Further reading

Kato GJ, et al. Sickle cell disease. *Nat Rev Dis Primers*, 2018;4:18010.

37. D

Total white cell count is increased in patients on corticosteroids. The effects on various classes of white blood cells are as follows:

- Polymorphonuclear leucocytes: Increased
- Lymphocytes: Decreased
- Monocytes and eosinophils: Decreased

Other causes of neutrophil leucocytosis include, i.e. abnormally high number of neutrophils include infections, inflammatory conditions, e.g. adult-onset rheumatoid arthritis, Crohn's disease, ulcerative colitis, chronic granulomatous infections, bronchiectasis, chronic myeloid leukaemia, polycythaemia vera, primary myelofibrosis, essential thrombocytosis, etc.

Anaemia, granulocytopaenia, and thrombocytopenia are not side effects and therefore incorrect. Lymphocyte count is decreased; therefore lymphocytosis is also not plausible. Neutrophils leucocytosis is the most plausible and correct option.

Further reading

Stanbury RM, Graham EM. Systemic corticosteroid therapy—side effects and their management. *Br J Ophthalmol*, 1998;82(6):704–8.

38. A

Acute lymphoblastic leukaemia (ALL) is a malignant transformation and proliferation of lymphoid progenitor cells in the bone marrow, blood, and extramedullary sites. There is abnormal proliferation and differentiation of a clonal population of lymphoid cells resulting in constitutional symptoms 'B symptoms' (fever, weight loss, night sweats) and signs of bone marrow failure (anaemia, thrombocytopenia, leukopenia) manifesting as easy bleeding or bruising, fatigue, dyspnoea, and infection. 80% of ALL occurs in children with a peak incidence between 0 and 4 in the UK.

Bone marrow failure would manifest as complete pancytopenia without any marked increase in white blood cell count.

Burkitt's lymphoma is a highly aggressive B-cell non-Hodgkin lymphoma which is associated with EBV. It has a chromosomal translocation that activates an oncogene (*c-MYC*). There are three clinical variants: endemic (associated with malaria), sporadic (the predominant type found in non-malarial areas), and immunodeficiency-related (HIV related). Sporadic Burkitt's lymphoma commonly present in the abdomen (60–80%), presenting symptoms include abdominal pain, distension, nausea and vomiting, and gastrointestinal bleeding. They can also present in the head and neck as lymphadenopathy. Endemic Burkitt's lymphoma most frequently present with jaw or periorbital swellings, or abdominal involvement (of retroperitoneal tissue, gut, ovary, or kidney). The jaw involvement is common in young children. Infiltration of the bone marrow is rare.

Chronic myeloid leukaemia is a myeloproliferative neoplasm involving a fusion of the Abelson gene (*ABL1*) from chromosome 9q34 with the breakpoint cluster region (BCR) gene on chromosome 22q11.2. This rearrangement is known as the Philadelphia chromosome. The molecular consequence of this translocation is the generation of a BCR-ABL1 fusion oncogene, which in turn translates into a BCR-ABL1 oncoprotein. It is an adult leukaemia with a peak incidence between 85 and 89 in the UK. It accounts for up to 15% of newly diagnosed cases of leukaemia in adults.

Acute myeloblastic leukaemia (AML) is characterized by infiltration of the bone marrow, blood, and other tissues by proliferative, clonal, abnormally differentiated, and occasionally poorly differentiated cells of the haematopoietic system. AML is the most common acute leukaemia in adults with a median age at presentation of 67 years and a peak incidence between 85 and 89 in the UK.

The signs and symptoms are suggestive of leukaemia, that is, a rapid accumulation of dysfunctional immature white blood cells which suppress the production of other cell lines producing signs of marrow failure. On the ground of age incidence, the most plausible option is ALL as 80% of cases occur in children. It is also the most common cancer in children.

Further reading

Cancer Research UK. Statistics by cancer type. Available at: https://www.cancerresearchuk.org/health-professional/cancer-statistics/statistics-by-cancer-type

Grigoropoulos NF, Petter R, Van't Veer MB, Scott MA, Follows GA. Leukaemia update. Part 1: diagnosis and management. *BMJ*, 2013;346:f1660.

39. A

Bleeding episodes post-surgery (extraction) are more likely to occur when the platelet count is low (i.e. $<20 \times 10^9/L$). To minimize the risk of postoperative bleeding a preoperative platelet level of $50 \times 10^9/L$ is advocated for minor surgery and $100 \times 10^9/L$ for more invasive surgery. For patients with significantly low platelet counts, this may need to be achieved by platelet transfusion prior to surgery. Studies have shown that post-extraction bleeding in patients with platelet count of $100 \times 10^9/L$ was infrequent and where present can be easily controlled with local measures such as primary closure via suturing, injection of vasoconstrictor locally, or application of one of a host of haemostatic materials: gelatine sponge (Gelfoam), oxidized regenerated cellulose (Surgicel), etc. into the socket.

In this patient, the platelet level is $100 \times 10^9/L$, therefore, a platelet transfusion is not required. While post-extraction bleeding is unlikely at this platelet level proceeding with the extraction as normal would be considered negligent. Tranexamic acid is an antifibrinolytic used to prevent the breakdown of blood clot, it has been studied extensively in the setting of dental extractions for patients at risk of bleeding (haemophilia), although not specifically in the thrombocytopenic patient. Oral corticosteroid therapy prior to the extraction would be beneficial if the patients had idiopathic thrombocytopenia. Therefore, the most likely recommendation would be to apply local haemostatic measures as just described to minimize post-extraction oozing.

Further reading

Fillmore WJ, Leavitt BD, Arce K. Dental extraction in the thrombocytopenic patient is safe and complications are easily managed. *J Oral Maxillofac Surg*, 2013;71(10):1647–52.

40. C

Plummer–Vinson (Paterson–Brown–Kelly) syndrome is rare and characterized by the triad of post-cricoid dysphagia, iron deficiency anaemia, and upper oesophageal webs. Historically it mainly affected white middle-aged women in the fourth to seventh decade of life. Clinical features resulting from anaemia include glossitis, angular cheilitis, koilonychia, weakness, fatigue, and tachycardia. Patients with Plummer–Vinson syndrome have an increased risk of developing squamous carcinoma of the oropharynx and oesophagus (post-cricoid area). Hence it is imperative these patients managed with iron supplementation and are followed-up closely. Plummer–Vinson syndrome can be managed effectively with iron supplementation and mechanical dilation.

Further reading

Novacek G. Plummer–Vinson syndrome. *Orphanet J Rare Dis*, 2006;1(1):36.

41. C

EBV is a gamma-herpes virus that infects >90% of normal adults through contact with oral secretions. Primary infection manifests as infectious mononucleosis. Post primary infection, the virus remains in an asymptomatic latent state within resting B-cells for the lifetime of the host. Cytotoxic T cells, both CD8+ and CD4+, and natural killer (NK) cells are primarily responsible for containing the infection. Under circumstances where the host's cellular immune system fails to control EBV-induced B-cell proliferation, infected carrier B-cells transform from their latent state into malignant cells as seen in EBV-associated lymphomas. EBV-associated lymphoma includes Burkitt's, Hodgkin and diffuse large B-cell lymphomas, and NK/T-cell lymphoma.

While all of the lymphomas in the option and infectious mononucleosis can be associated with EBV infection and constitutional B symptoms (fatigue, weight loss, night sweats), the nodular architecture and presence of Reed–Sternberg cells (the malignant cells) is characteristic of Hodgkin's lymphoma. The Hodgkin Reed–Sternberg (HRS) cells are large, binucleated tumour cells. Therefore, the most plausible cause of the patient's neck lymph node swelling is Hodgkin's lymphoma.

Further reading

Roschewski M, Wilson WH. EBV-associated lymphomas in adults. *Best Pract Res Clin Haematol*, 2012;25(1):75–89.

Special investigations in relation to medicine in dentistry

42. D

The signs and symptoms described are indicative of haematological malignancies. Therefore, all of the options are plausible at this point. Genetic changes in leukaemic cells are well established as the drivers of tumour growth.

In chronic myeloid leukaemia, the Philadelphia chromosome caused by translocation of genetic material between chromosomes 9 and 22 giving rise to a shorter than normal chromosome 22. This translocation gives rise fusion of the Abelson gene (*ABL1*) from chromosome 9q34 with the *BCR* gene on chromosome 22q11.2. The molecular consequence of this translocation is the generation of a BCR-ABL1 fusion oncogene, which in turn translates into a BCR-ABL1 oncoprotein. This oncoprotein cause constitutive induction of the ABL1 tyrosine kinase pathway resulting autonomous proliferation of malignant myeloid cells.

In Burkitt's lymphoma, the translocation t(8;14)(q24;q32) is the hallmark and occurs in 70–80% of patients. The variant translocations, t(2;8)(p12;q24) and t(8;22)(q24;q11), occur in 10–15% of patients. The molecular consequence of this translocation is deregulated expression of the *MYC* oncogene, which has an essential role in cell cycle control. Again, the consequence is autonomous proliferation of the lymphoma cells.

In ALL, characteristic translocations which include t(12;21) [*ETV6-RUNX1*], t(1;19) [*TCF3-PBX1*], t(9;22) [*BCR-ABL1*] and rearrangement of *MLL* are noted.

In chronic lymphocytic leukaemia, 80% of patients carry at least one of four common chromosomal alterations: a deletion in chromosome 13q14.3 (del(13q)), del(11q), del(17p), and trisomy 12. The consequence of this is prolonged cell survival due to inhibition of apoptosis and autonomous/uninhibited cell cycle progression.

In Hodgkin's lymphoma, because of the small number of malignant cells, cytogenetic analysis is particularly difficult, hence no specific chromosomal rearrangements have been detected to date.

Therefore, the most plausible option is chronic myeloid leukaemia because of its consistent association with the Philadelphia chromosome.

Further reading

Wilkinson IB, Raine T, Wiles K, Goodhart A, Hall C, O'Neill H. Chapter 8: Haematology. In: Wilkinson IB, *et al.* (eds). *Oxford Handbook of Clinical Medicine*, 10th Edition. Oxford, UK: Oxford University Press, 2019.

43. B

Causes of macroglossia include:

- Hypothyroidism
- Acromegaly
- Granular cell tumour
- Idiopathic muscular hypertrophy
- Beckwith–Wiedemann syndrome
- Amyloidosis

Histological confirmation of amyloid through Congo red staining producing apple-green birefringence under cross-polarized light as seen in this patient remains the diagnostic gold standard. Therefore, the most plausible option is amyloidosis.

However, elucidating the pathophysiology responsible for the type of amyloidosis this patient is likely to deposit is a good knowledge to have. A brief outline of the classification of amyloidosis would facilitate this.

Amyloidosis can be acquired or inherited and there about 20 different proteins that can form amyloid fibrils *in vivo*. Three common types of amyloidosis:

- Serum amyloid A protein (AA)- reactive systemic amyloidosis and is associated with chronic inflammatory states
- Monoclonal immunoglobulin light chain (AL)-systemic amyloidosis associated with monoclonal plasma cell dyscrasias
- β_2 microglobulin (Aβ2M)-periarticular and occasionally systemic amyloidosis associated with long-term dialysis

In this patient, the longstanding bronchiectasis (irreversible dilation of bronchi due to destruction of the bronchial walls) evident by bronchial destruction on chest radiograph is a chronic inflammatory disease. The association between chronic inflammatory disease and secondary amyloidosis has long been recognized. Therefore, in bronchiectasis, where there is sustained acute phase response, deposition of reactive systemic, AA, amyloidosis is a potential complication. In fact, bronchiectasis is the major respiratory disease underlying secondary AA amyloidosis and accounting for 5% of cases in the UK. Other purely respiratory causes of AA amyloidosis are tuberculosis, the commonest single disease resulting in AA amyloid in many parts of the developing world. Other less common associations include cystic fibrosis, sarcoidosis, and Kartagener's syndrome. Secondary AA amyloidosis irrespective of the underlying pathology is characterized by the deposition of AA-type amyloid in multiple organs and tissues of the body, the tongue inclusive.

Further reading

Lachmann HJ, Hawkins PN. Amyloidosis and the lung. *Chron Respir Dis*, 2006;3(4):203–14.

44. A

The signs and symptoms described are indicative of marrow failure due to acute leukaemia. Eighty per cent (80%) of children with acute leukaemia have ALL, the remaining 20% acute myeloid leukaemia. In acute leukaemia, genetic mutation in blood progenitor cells leads to developmental arrest of progenitor cells at a particular point in their differentiation and uncontrollable capacity for self-renewal. The resultant effect is the body is overwhelmed by immature cells or blasts that infiltrate the bone marrow, reticulo-endothelial system, and other extramedullary sites. Other pathophysiological processes include systemic effects of cytokines produced by the blast cells. Signs and symptoms on the basis of the three main pathological processes listed earlier can be seen in Table 2.6.

Table 2.6 Pathophysiological processes in acute leukaemia and their corresponding clinical manifestations

Pathophysiological process	Signs and symptoms
Systemic effects of cytokines	Malaise, fatigue, nausea, fever
Bone marrow infiltration	Anaemia (pallor, lethargy, shortness of breath, palpitation, dizziness) Neutropenia (fever, infections, opportunistic infections like oral candidiasis) Thrombocytopenia (petechiae, epistaxis, bruising)
Reticuloendothelial system	Hepatosplenomegaly Lymphadenopathy
Gingiva	Gingiva hypertrophy

Special investigations and corresponding findings:

- Full blood count and differentials will show pancytopenia, neutropenia, and overall raised white cell count secondary to numerous circulating blasts.
- Blood film (peripheral blood smear)—Blast may be seen in peripheral circulation hence clearly evident on the film. In other cases, blasts remain sequestered in the bone marrow resulting in the absence of clearly identifiable blasts in blood films.
- Coagulation profile—With the exception of BT which will be prolonged because of thrombocytopenia, the other coagulation tests (INR, PT, and APTT) are expected to be within normal range.
- Serum electrophoresis—This is not of diagnostic use in acute leukaemia because no abnormal serum proteins are produced in excess.
- Bone marrow biopsy or aspirate—This is obtained under general anaesthesia in children, this test provides morphological, immunological, and genetic information, which allows for establishing a definitive diagnosis.

Other tests utilized include flow cytometry for assessing the immunophenotype of subtypes of particular acute leukaemia and cytogenetic analysis to identify specific genetic abnormalities, which may be of prognostic importance.

In summary, an abnormal full blood count, peripheral blood film, prolonged BT in conjunction with a suspicious clinical picture should prompt urgent referral to a tertiary care centre for a bone marrow biopsy, the most helpful in establishing a definitive diagnosis in this 9-year-old boy.

Further reading

Mitchell C, Hall G, Clarke RT. Acute leukaemia in children: diagnosis and management. *BMJ*, 2009;338:b2285.

Wilkinson IB, Raine T, Wiles K, Goodhart A, Hall C, O'Neill H. Chapter 8: Haematology. In: Wilkinson IB, *et al.* (eds). *Oxford Handbook of Clinical Medicine*, 10th Edition. Oxford, UK: Oxford University Press, 2019.

45. C

Hypercalcaemia is diagnosed when the concentration of serum calcium is two standard deviations above the mean of values found in people with normal calcium levels, in at least two samples at least 1 week apart over a period of 3 months. The serum concentration of total calcium in adults usually ranges between 2.15 and 2.60 mmol/L.

Cause of hypercalcaemia include:

- Parathyroid hormone mediated:
  - Primary hyperthyroidism (parathyroid adenoma, hyperplasia, or carcinoma)
  - Tertiary hyperparathyroidism
  - Ectopic parathyroid producing malignancy
  - Familial hypocalciuric hypercalcaemia
- Non-parathyroid hormone mediated/malignancy associated:
  - Overproduction of parathyroid hormone-related peptide by tumour cells (humoral hypercalcaemia of malignancy)
  - Excess conversion of vitamin D to active 1,25-dihydroxyvitamin D by lymphomas that leads to increased intestinal calcium absorption (absorptive hypercalcaemia)
  - Bone dissolution by metastasis or MM through secretion of local parathyroid hormone-related protein (PTHrP), cytokine, and chemokines (local osteolysis)

- Vitamin D related:
  - ◆ Granulomatous disease (sarcoidosis, tuberculosis, etc.)
  - ◆ Vitamin D intoxication
- Drugs:
  - ◆ Lithium
  - ◆ Thiazide diuretics
  - ◆ Milk-alkali syndrome
  - ◆ Vitamin A intoxication
- Miscellaneous:
  - ◆ Immobilization
  - ◆ Acute renal failure

The occurrence of hypercalcaemia together with systemic symptoms (for example, polydipsia, depression, abdominal pain, worsening malaise, lethargy, fever, weight loss, decreased appetite, etc.) should raise suspicion of malignancy. Hypercalcaemia is usually a late finding in malignancy. In this patient, the presence of monoclonal light chain paraprotein band detected on serum and urinary electrophoresis is characteristic of MM.

If the primary malignancy was unknown a comprehensive history (including review of medications), physical examination (including lymph nodes, rectal, breasts, gynaecological, mouth, and ear, nose, and throat), extensive laboratory assessment (blood count, biochemistry, serum tumour markers), imaging (CT and MRI), and serum and urine electrophoresis would be required to arrive at a definitive diagnosis.

Based on the aforementioned discussion, the most plausible option is MM.

Further reading

BMJ Best Practice. Assessment of hypercalcaemia. Available at: https://www.bestpractice.bmj.com/best-practice/monograph/159.html

Minisola S, Pepe J, Piemonte S, Cipriani C. The diagnosis and management of hypercalcaemia. *BMJ*, 2015;350:h2723.

46. B

Acute hypocalcaemia can be life-threatening. Patients can become symptomatic when the threshold drops below 1.9 mmol/L.

Clinical features of acute hypocalcaemia:

- Perioral and digital paraesthesia
- Positive Trousseau's and Chvostek's signs
- Tetany and carpel tunnel spasms
- Laryngospasm
- Electrocardiograph (ECG) changes (prolonged QT interval) and arrhythmia
- Seizures

Causes of hypocalcaemia:

- Severe vitamin D deficiency
- Selective parathyroidectomy (hypocalcaemia is mild and transient)
- Magnesium deficiency
- Disruption of parathyroid gland function due to total thyroidectomy

- Cytotoxic drug-induced hypocalcaemia
- Pancreatitis, rhabdomyolysis, and large volume blood transfusions

Among the list of options, three are plausible causes of hypocalcaemia they include hypomagnesaemia, hypoparathyroidism, and vitamin D deficiency. Hypothyroidism and postoperative critical illness are not likely causes, therefore not options to be considered. Considering this patient has just undergone a total thyroidectomy, where disruption to parathyroid gland function is a complication. The most plausible option is hypoparathyroidism. In fact, disruption of the parathyroid gland function due to total thyroidectomy is the most common cause of acute symptomatic hypocalcaemia in hospital practice.

Management: If post-thyroidectomy and patient asymptomatic, repeat calcium 24 h later:

- When adjusted calcium is >2.1 mmol/L, patient may be discharged and recheck calcium within 1 week
- If serum calcium remains between 1.9 and 2.1 mmol/L, increase sandocal 1,000 to three BD
- If patient remains in mild hypocalcaemic range beyond 72 h postoperatively despite calcium supplementation, start alfacalcidol 0.25 µg/day with close monitoring

Further reading

Turner J, Gittoes N, Selby P, Society for Endocrinology Clinical Committee. Society for endocrinology endocrine emergency guidance: emergency management of acute hypocalcaemia in adult patients. *Endocr Connect*, 2016;5(5):G7.

47. E

The clinical presentation of the patient in this scenario, i.e. weight gain, cold intolerance, fatigue, mood impairment (depression and flat affects) are indicative of hypothyroidism. Other clinical features of hypothyroidism include fatigue on exertion, hoarseness of voice, constipation, menstrual disturbance, muscle weakness and cramp, dry coarse skin, hair loss (loss of lateral eyebrows). Hypothyroidism increases total cholesterol, low-density lipoprotein, and homocysteine concentrations. The implications for these patients are they may present with features of metabolic syndrome including hypertension, increased waist circumference, and dyslipidaemia. Their dyslipidaemia can manifest as yellowish plaque deposits around the eyelids which are referred to as xanthelasma.

Increased high density lipoprotein (HDL) and low TSH levels, increased low-density lipoprotein (LDL) and low thyroxine (T4) levels are close options. However, low TSH levels will lead to increased thyroxine levels via the feedback mechanism, therefore not a plausible option. The most plausible option is therefore increased LDL and low thyroxine (T4) levels.

Further reading

Chaker L, Bianco AC, Jonklass J, Peters RP. Hypothyroidism. *Lancet*, 2017; 390(10101):1550–62.

48. A

The patient clinical features including the mucocutaneous pigmentation should raise the suspicion for AD. Therefore, an urgent referral to the endocrinologist to establish a definitive diagnosis and manage is critical as AD can be fatal if not treated.

AD, also known as primary adrenal insufficiency and secondary adrenal insufficiency, can present similar features with the exception of mucocutaneous hyperpigmentation which is characteristic of the former. In both settings, an adrenal crisis, can occur following significant stress or illness, however, this is more likely to happen in primary adrenal insufficiency. The clinical features and investigation findings are attributable to cortisol and aldosterone deficiency, and excess ACTH which is seen only in AD.

Cortisol deficiency—Weakness, fatigue, weight loss, anorexia progressing to nausea, vomiting, diarrhoea, abdominal pain, and low blood glucose levels.

Aldosterone deficiency—Hyponatraemia, hyperkalaemia, acidosis, tachycardia, and hypotension. Suggestive symptoms are postural hypotension and salt cravings.

Excess ACTH is only present in primary adrenal insufficiency. The excess ACTH levels from the pituitary gland results in a corresponding increase in α-melanocyte-stimulating hormone. Both hormones stimulate the melanocortin 1 receptor on keratinocytes to promote melanogenesis and thus the characteristic mucocutaneous pigmentation. In the oral cavity this can manifest as patchy melanosis affecting multiple locations including the vermillion border of the lips and buccal mucosa.

Investigation findings:

- Serum electrolyte levels may show hyponatraemia and hyperkalaemia
- A low serum cortisol level at 8 a.m. suggests adrenal insufficiency. Random serum cortisol level is not diagnostic as the levels fluctuate throughout the day in a diurnal pattern and with stress
- Raised plasma renin level and reduced serum aldosterone level

These special investigations, although out of range, do not distinguish between primary and secondary adrenal insufficiency.

Dexamethasone suppression test is used to measure adrenal gland function by assessing cortisol levels change in response to administration of dexamethasone. It is used to establish a diagnosis of Cushing's syndrome.

Adrenocortical hormone stimulation (ACTH) test, also known as Synacthen's test or cosyntropin stimulation test, is the first-line test for diagnosing primary adrenal insufficiency (AD). It can also be used to differentiate between primary and secondary adrenal insufficiency. In this test, serum cortisol, plasma ACTH, plasma aldosterone, and plasma renin levels are measured before administering 250 mcg of ACTH. At 30 and 60 minutes after intravenous ACTH administration, the serum cortisol levels are measured again. A normal response occurs with peak cortisol levels greater than 18–20 mcg per dl. A smaller or absent response is diagnostic for adrenal insufficiency. If there is impaired cortisol response, and ACTH >200 ng/L (i.e. low cortisol and high ACTH), then diagnosis is primary adrenal insufficiency. If ACTH <10 ng/L (i.e. low cortisol and low ACTH), then the diagnosis is secondary adrenal insufficiency.

Further special investigations include measurement of 21-hydroxylase antibody levels specific for identifying autoimmune adrenalitis. Computed tomography imaging of the adrenal gland to assess for other adrenal gland pathology (i.e. neoplasm or infections, i.e. tuberculosis).

Therefore, adrenocortical hormone stimulation (ACTH) test is the most helpful special investigation required to establish a definitive diagnosis of primary adrenal insufficiency (AD).

Further reading

Michels A, Michels N. Addison disease early detection and treatment principles. *Am Fam Physician*, 2014;89(7):563–8.

O'Connell S, Siafarikas A. Addison disease: diagnosis and initial management. *Aust Fam Physician*, 2010;39(11):834.

49. A

The patient presents several risk factors for osteoporosis, they include age, Asian race, smoking, postmenopausal status, low body weight, and the imminent commencement of steroid treatment. Considering her numerous risk factors, routine monitoring of her bone mineral density must be instituted to assess for osteoporosis, the risk of pathological fracture and potential side effects of the steroid treatment for pemphigus vulgaris. Diagnostic imaging tests that can be used to measure bone mineral density are CT scans, X-rays, ultrasound, and dual-energy X-ray absorptiometry (DEXA) scan. A bone profile blood test (calcium, phosphate, alkaline phosphatase, vitamin D) is usually normal in osteoporosis, but may be elevated in other bone disease. Hormone profile blood tests can be useful for detecting underlying disease that can have an effect on bone health (e.g. parathyroid hormone to check for hyperparathyroidism, thyroid hormones for thyroid disease, etc.).

Bone mineral density (BMD) is the primary test used to identify osteoporosis and low bone mass. The most preferred and accurate way for assessing BMD is DEXA scan. DEXA is performed on the central skeleton to measure the BMD of the lumbar spine and hip.

There are advantages of DEXA scans compared to other imaging test used to assess for BMD (i.e. ultrasound, X-ray, CT scan are short scan time, low radiation dose, rapid patient set up, good precision, consensus that BMD results can be interpreted using WHO T-scores). Furthermore, DEXA scans are non-invasive, inexpensive, and have been proven to be clinically useful to monitor patients treated for osteoporosis. Therefore, BMD measurement by DEXA scan is the most plausible option.

Further reading

South-Paul JE, Talabi MB. Chapter 30: Osteoporosis. In: South-Paul JE (ed.). *Current Diagnosis & Treatment in Family Medicine*, 4th Edition. New York, USA: McGraw-Hill Education/Medical, 2015.

50. B

Vitamin D is a fat-soluble vitamin utilized by the body for normal bone development and absorption of calcium, magnesium, and phosphate.

Causes of vitamin D deficiency are:

- Dietary deficiency
- Inadequate exposure to sunlight
- Malabsorption syndromes like coeliac disease, short bowel syndrome, IBD, etc.
- Chronic liver
- Chronic kidney
- Post-surgical hypothyroidism
- Medications

The chronic kidney disease in this patient means there is failure of enzymatic hydroxylation step resulting in vitamin D deficiency and consequently hypocalcaemia.

The hallmark of acute hypocalcaemia is neuromuscular irritability. Clinical features include numbness and tingling in the perioral region, fingertips and toes, paraesthesia, muscle cramps, fatigue, anxiety, etc. Clinically, neuromuscular irritability can be demonstrated by eliciting Chvostek's or Trousseau's signs.

Battle's sign is defined by retroauricular or mastoid ecchymosis that is typically the result of basilar skull fracture.

Chvostek's sign is elicited by tapping the skin over the facial nerve anterior to the external auditory meatus. Ipsilateral contraction of the facial muscles occurs in individuals with hypocalcaemia. Chvostek's sign is also present in 10% of normal individuals.

Nikolsky's sign describes the observation that a shearing force, such as when using a finger to laterally pull on the skin surrounding a lesion, will result in the separation of the epidermis and creation of an erosion. It is a sign consistent with blistering mucocutaneous abnormalities.

Russell's sign is defined as calluses on the knuckles or back of the hand due to repeated self-induced vomiting over long periods of time. The condition is brought about from the afflicted person's knuckles making contact with the incisor teeth during the act of inducing the gag reflex at the back of the throat with their finger(s). It is primarily found in patients with an eating disorder such as bulimia nervosa or anorexia nervosa.

Trousseau's sign is elicited by inflation of a blood pressure cuff to 20 mmHg above the patient's systolic blood pressure for 3–5 minutes. Carpal spasm presents as flexion of the wrist and of the metacarpal phalangeal joints, extension of the interphalangeal joints, and abduction of the thumb.

Chvostek's sign best describes this patient's findings (i.e. spasms of facial muscles elicited by tapping the skin over the facial nerve anterior to the external auditory meatus). Therefore, it is the most plausible option.

Further reading

Schafer AL, Shoback DM. Hypocalcemia: diagnosis and treatment. In: Feingold KR, *et al.* (eds). *Endotext [Internet]*. South Dartmouth (MA): MDText. Com, Inc, 2016.

Medical emergencies in dentistry

51. E

Long-term exogenous glucocorticoid (prednisolone) use is a common cause of adrenal insufficiency. Patient with adrenal insufficiency carry a significant risk of developing an adrenal crisis particularly when faced with a precipitating event. Precipitating events include surgical stress, physical stress/pain, emotional stress, all of which can be experienced during dental treatment. This risk of developing an adrenal crisis is higher in primary compared to secondary adrenal insufficiency due to lack of mineralocorticoid and a greater risk of dehydration and hypovolaemia. In glucocorticoid induced adrenal insufficiency, this risk also exists but difficult to determine precisely. Patients with adrenal crisis develop hypotension and may have altered sensorium and even collapse, as is the case in this scenario. The hypotension is due to hypovolaemia and hypercortisolism. They can also present abdominal pain, nausea, vomiting, and diarrhoea leading to an erroneous diagnosis of an acute abdomen and gastroenteritis. Hypoglycaemia and hyponatraemia are likely biochemical features.

In the event of a crisis, the principles of therapy are fluid resuscitation and steroid replacement. Fluid resuscitation with isotonic sodium chloride 0.9% will correct the hypovolaemia and hyponatraemia and intravenous dextrose to correct hypoglycaemia. Steroid replacement administered intravenously or intramuscularly as 100 mg bolus every 6 hours until recovery. As both principles of therapy are best administered in a hospital setting, the initial management in a dental setting should aim to minimize effect of the hypotensive episode by laying the patient flat, giving oxygen, and arranging urgent transfer to the hospital where fluid resuscitation and corticosteroid replacement can be commenced. In the future, prior to treating patient on long-term prednisolone, the dentist should consider increasing their glucocorticoid dose (under the guidance of the patient's GP or endocrinologist) to cover for the stress induced by receiving dental treatment.

Further reading

Jevon P. Updated posters to help manage medical emergencies in the dental practice. *Br Dent J*, 2015;219(5):227.

Puar TH, Stikkelbroeck NM, Smans LC, Zelissen PM, Hermus AR. Adrenal crisis: still a deadly event in the 21st century. *Am J Med*, 2016;129(3):339.e1–9.

52. B

Hypoglycaemia is a lower than normal level of blood glucose. It can be defined as 'mild' if the episode is self-treated and 'severe' if assistance by a third party is required. Clinical features include sweating, palpitation, shaking, hunger, confusion, drowsiness, aggressive behaviour, speech difficulty, nausea, headache, etc. Causes of hypoglycaemia include missed or delayed meals, inappropriately timed insulin, or oral hypoglycaemic therapy in relation to meal, increased exercise (relative to usual), etc.

Orthostatic hypotension refers to the development of symptoms such as light-headedness and blurred vision when a subject stands up that clears on sitting back down or on prolonged standing. It can also be defined by a drop-in blood pressure of at least 20 mmHg for systolic blood pressure and at least 10 mmHg for diastolic blood pressure within 3 minutes of standing up. These symptoms are due to cerebral hypoperfusion. Risk factors for orthostatic hypotension include age (elderly), multiple medications, smoking status, low body mass index, hypertension (treated or not), and diabetes. Medications particularly antihypertensive drugs are the most intuitive culprits especially in the elderly. They include beta blockers (bisoprolol), alpha blockers (prazosin), and diuretics (spironolactone and bendroflumethiazide). Calcium channel blockers (amlodipine) and angiotensin receptor antagonists (valsartan) are also culprits but less associated with orthostatic hypotension compared to sympathomimetic drugs. The number of antihypertensive drugs used has been reported as predictive of orthostatic hypotension.

Vasovagal syncope occurs when an otherwise normal person with normal baroreceptor reflexes suddenly faints. It can be triggered by pain or emotional stimulus and usually result in abrupt fall in blood pressure accompanied by a similarly abrupt fall in heart rate (patient sudden collapse and fall to the ground).

Pseudo syncope (psychogenic syncope) is the appearance of transient loss of consciousness in the absence of true loss of consciousness. In the most recent syncope guidelines, it was defined as a syndrome of apparent loss of consciousness occurring in the absence of impaired cerebral perfusion or function. It is associated with psychological stresses, that is, a conversion disorder

Vertigo is the hallucination of movement of the environment around the patient, or of the patient with respect to the environment. Vertigo is not the same as dizziness. Rather dizziness is a non-specific term which can be categorized into four different subtypes (i.e. vertigo, light-headedness, presyncope, and disequilibrium). Vertigo can either be peripheral (i.e. due to disorders of the inner ear or the vestibulocochlear (eighth) cranial nerve), or central (i.e. due to a brainstem or cerebellar disorder).

Considering this patient is elderly and on multiple antihypertensive drugs, the most likely culprit for the light-headedness on standing up is orthostatic hypotension.

Further reading

Joseph A, Wanono R, Flamant M, Vidal-Petiot E. Orthostatic hypotension: a review. *Nephrol Ther*, 2017;13:S55–67.

53. B

A reaction following parenteral penicillin administration and the patient's clinical features are indicative of an anaphylactic reaction. Administration of 0.5 ml of 1:1,000 (500 μg) adrenaline via intramuscularly route is the first-line management for an anaphylactic reaction. The dose is repeated if necessary, at 5-minute intervals according to blood pressure, pulse, and respiratory function of the patient until there is resolution of anaphylaxis or signs of toxicity occur. Irrespective of the initial recovery, a second anaphylactic (biphasic) reaction can occur after an asymptomatic period of up to 72 hours with most occurring within the first 8 hours. For this reason, patients must be transferred to hospital irrespective of their initial recovery.

Adrenaline is a sympathomimetic catecholamine. It acts on alpha-adrenergic receptors to lessen peripheral vasodilation and increased vascular permeability both of which causes loss of intravascular fluid volume and hypotension. On beta-adrenergic receptors, it exerts bronchodilatory effects via β_2 receptors located on airway smooth muscles causing bronchial smooth muscle relaxation. This alleviates bronchospasm, wheezing, and dyspnoea. The beta-adrenergic action also increases the force of myocardial contraction to enhance coronary blood flow and increase cardiac output and blood pressure.

Antihistamines and steroids are both second-line management of anaphylactic reaction.

Oxygen should be given as soon as available.

β_2 agonists are used for management of shortness of breath associated with acute asthmatic attacks. Their bronchodilatory effects are meditated via β_2 receptors located on airway smooth muscles. Examples of β_2 agonists include salbutamol, terbutaline, salmeterol, etc.

Therefore, the most important class of medication for acute management of the patient's medical emergency (anaphylaxis) is catecholamines.

Further reading

Resuscitation Council UK. *Guidance: Anaphylaxis.* Available at: https://www.resus.org.uk/anaphylaxis/emergency-treatment-of-anaphylactic-reactions/

54. C

The patient is experiencing a precipitate asthmatic attack triggered by psychological stress from the post-extraction pain and the use of naproxen, a NSAID.

Predictors from the medical history of an increased likelihood of developing an asthmatic attack are as follows:

- History of a recent severe asthma exacerbation;
- History of emergency department visit or hospitalization for asthma in the prior year;
- History of the amount of short-acting β_2-agonists (SABA) self-administered during an asthmatic attack. Daily short-acting β_2-agonists (SABAs) reflect very poorly controlled asthma and is associated with increased risk of acute exacerbations. Extrapolating the amount of SABA used can also be helpful too, studies have shown that the use of more than three canisters of SABA in the past 3 months implies daily use which correlates with poorly controlled asthma;
- History of asthmatic attack following smoking;
- History of upper or lower respiratory tract infection;
- History of poor compliance with long-term control medications such as inhaled corticosteroids;
- History of allergen or pollutant exposure.

History of daily use of inhaled corticosteroids and history of use of no more than one salbutamol inhaler canister in the preceding 3 months are both indicators of well controlled asthma, therefore not plausible option.

Although asthma and atopy have a causal relationship, they are separate entities and are inherited separately, therefore a history of parental atopy is not a direct predictor of developing an asthmatic attack particularly in adults.

There are no reports of correlation between food allergy and the risk of developing an asthmatic attack. That said, a severe asthmatic attack associated with other anaphylactic symptoms can occur following the ingestion of an offending food.

A history of recent upper or lower respiratory tract infection is the most useful predictor of the risk of developing an asthmatic attack in this patient. Administration of NSAID can further exacerbate this risk by resulting in the generation of leukotriene, a potent constrictor of bronchial smooth muscles. This is thought to be as a result of diversion of arachidonic acid metabolism to the 5-lipoxygenase pathway following inhibition of the cyclooxygenase enzyme.

Further reading

Fergeson JE, Patel SS, Lockey RF. Acute asthma, prognosis, and treatment. *J Allergy Clin Immunol,* 2017;139(2):438–47.

55. A

The patient is experiencing a cerebrovascular attack (stroke) based on the clinical features presented. Strokes can be broadly divided into ischaemic or haemorrhagic with majority being ischaemic (~80%). The risk factors can be subdivided into modifiable and non-modifiable, and are as follows:

- Modifiable:
  - Hypertension
  - Hyperlipidaemia
  - Current smoking
  - Waist-to-hip ratio
  - Diet
  - Alcohol consumption
  - Diabetes
  - AF and atrial cardiopathy
  - Physical inactivity
  - Genetics
- Non-modifiable:
  - Age
  - Sex
  - Race/ethnicity
  - Genetics

All of the options can be aetiologically associated with a stroke either directly or indirectly as shown next.

Hormonal factors such as oral contraceptive use, pregnancy, post-partum state are risk factors for developing stroke in women at a younger age.

Hypothyroidism is associated with increase total cholesterol, LDL, and homocysteine concentrations. The implications are patients can present with features of metabolic syndrome including hypertension, increased waist circumference, and dyslipidaemia, all of which are risk factors for stroke.

Sickle cell disease exhibits an autosomal recessive mode of inheritance and is caused by a mutation in chromosome 11 that results in the replacement of glutamic acid with valine at position 6 of the N-terminus of the globin chain. Patients can present large and small vessel disease putting them at risk of developing an ischaemic stroke.

All NSAIDs, to some degree can affect vasoconstriction and sodium excretion, which can lead to hypertension, a risk factor for stroke. Potential mechanisms for this include vasoconstriction secondary to inhibition of prostacyclin induced vasodilation, hypertension induced by direct effects on sodium excretion leading to volume expansion and thrombosis due to prostaglandin mediated platelet aggregation. The stroke risk is thought to be dependent on a specific NSAID and the duration of use. For example, naproxen is thought to be associated with the highest increase in blood pressure, likewise chronic NSAID use.

Atrial fibrillation—The association between AF and stroke is thought to be due to stasis of blood in the fibrillating left atrium causing thrombus formation and embolization to the brain.

Considering 80% of strokes are ischaemic, the incidence of ischaemic stroke is higher in the elderly as there is no mention of any specific comorbidity in the question, the most likely option to be aetiologically associated with this patient stroke is AF. Atrial fibrillation is a risk factor for cardioembolic type of ischaemic stroke and studies have shown one-third of patients do not show evidence of AF until after a stroke despite months of preceding continuous heart-rhythm monitoring (i.e. it can be a silent disease).

Further reading

Boehme AK, Esenwa C, Elkind MS. Stroke risk factors, genetics, and prevention. *Circ Res*, 2017;120(3):472–95.

56. B

All of the following with the exception of option B should not feature in the policy for management of medical emergencies in dentistry. See the following guidelines, which should feature in this policy:

- All clinical dental staff (dentists, dental therapists, and dental nurses) and receptionists based within the clinics should undergo mandatory resuscitation training and use of an automated external defibrillator (AED).
- Medical history should be taken from all new patients attending the dental practice and all patients commencing a new course of dental treatment. Medical histories should also be updated at every check-up and whenever the practice is informed of a change of status in the patient's medical history.
- Medical emergencies drugs and equipment should be immediately available and accessible for use.
- Resuscitation equipment including AED and emergency drugs must be checked weekly.
- All dental staff should know how to call for emergency help using standard emergency call information which would facilitate correct details to be provided to the emergency services.
- Emergency drugs excluding oxygen should only be given by dentists who are trained in recognizing signs and symptoms of common medical emergencies in dentistry.

Further reading

Jevon P. Updated posters to help manage medical emergencies in the dental practice. *Br Dent J*, 2015;219(5):227.

57. E

The patient's clinical features are in keeping with orthostatic hypotension.

Orthostatic hypotension refers to the development of symptoms such as light-headedness and blurred vision when a subject stands up that clears on sitting back down or on prolonged standing. It can also be defined by a drop-in blood pressure of at least 20 mmHg for systolic blood pressure and at least 10 mmHg for diastolic blood pressure within 3 minutes of standing up. These symptoms are due to cerebral hypoperfusion. Risk factors for orthostatic hypotension include age (elderly), multiple medications, smoking status, low body mass index, hypertension (treated or not), and diabetes. Medications particularly antihypertensive drugs are the most intuitive culprits especially in the elderly. They include beta blockers (bisoprolol), alpha blockers (prazosin, tamsulosin), and diuretics (spironolactone and bendroflumethiazide). Calcium channel blockers (amlodipine) and angiotensin receptor antagonists (Valsartan) are also culprits but less associated with orthostatic hypotension compared to sympathomimetic drugs. Other factors include diabetics with autonomic neuropathy. In some cases, it could be idiopathic.

All of the medications in the option are used to manage the patient's comorbidities specifically metformin, a biguanide for type 2 diabetes, aspirin, and clopidogrel, both antiplatelets used to manage the patient's cardiovascular risk related to type 2 diabetes and simvastatin for management of hypercholesterolaemia, also a risk associated with being diabetic. Tamsulosin is a long-acting alpha blocker that relaxes the muscles in the bladder neck and prostrate. It is used to manage lower urinary tract symptoms (i.e. poor urinary stream and urinary frequency in men with enlarged prostrate).

Tamsulosin, an alpha-adrenergic blocker, is the most likely culprit for this patient's orthostatic hypotension. It lowers blood pressure resulting in unsteadiness or transient loss of consciousness and light-headedness on standing from supine position or following prolonged periods of standing. This effect can be particularly pronounced in elderly males who may have inadequate vasomotor reflexes for the various reasons highlighted here.

Further reading

Sathyapalan T, Aye MM, Atkin SL. Postural hypotension. *BMJ*, 2011;342:d3128.

58. B

A cerebrovascular accident or stroke is the sudden cessations of blood flow to areas of the brain leading to cell death. Strokes fall into two aetiologic categories: ischaemic or haemorrhagic. Ischaemic strokes are the sudden interruption of blood flow to the brain which can be due to thrombi, emboli, or compression. Haemorrhagic strokes are characterized by bleeding into the brain due to rupture of a blood vessel. Cerebrovascular accident or stroke causes upper motor neuron lesion. Upper motor neuron (UMN) lesions manifest as lower facial weakness and hemiparesis. A unique characteristic of UMN lesion is its tendency to affect specific muscle groups (i.e. in the face), facial weakness does not affect the forehead, since the neurones to the upper face receive bilateral UMN innervation. In other words, an UMN lesion is characterized by contralateral facial palsy, some sparing of the frontalis and orbicularis oculi muscles, spontaneous facial movements with emotional responses.

In contrast, lower motor neurone lesions produce full ipsilateral hemifacial weakness, including the forehead. Other features in lower motor neurone lesion are hyperacusis (due to loss of function of nerve to stapedius), loss of taste (due to loss of function to chorda tympani which supply special taste sensation to the anterior two-thirds of the tongue) and changes in lacrimation and salivation.

Painful rash over the ear is characteristic of Ramsay Hunt syndrome, which is defined as peripheral facial nerve palsy (lower motor neurone lesion) accompanied by an erythematous vesicular rash on the ear (zoster oticus) or in the mouth.

The most likely clinical feature from the list of options to characterize a cerebrovascular accident is furrowing of the brow, for the reasons highlighted earlier.

Further reading

Boehme AK, Esenwa C, Elkind MS. Stroke risk factors, genetics, and prevention. *Circ Res*, 2017;120(3):472–95.

Scully C. Sensory and motor changes. In: Scully C, et al. (eds). *Oral and Maxillofacial Medicine-E-Book: The Basis of Diagnosis and Treatment*. London, UK: Elsevier Health Sciences, 2012.

59. B

Epileptic seizures can occur in a dental practice. Patients usually experience sudden collapse and loss of consciousness, rigidity, and cyanosis, jerking movement of limb, noisy breathing, frothing at the mouth, incontinence, and accidental injuries; for example, tongue biting. Epileptic seizures are managed using 'ABCDE' refers to airway, breathing, circulation, disability, and exposure as is the case with all medical emergencies in dentistry. During the seizure attacks ensure the environment is safe to prevent injury, do not restrain or put anything in the patient's mouth. Note timing of the fit, once jerking movements cease give oxygen 15/minutes, place in the recovery position, and check airway.

It recommended calling the emergency helpline '999' if:

- Seizure persists for more than 5 minutes after emergency medication has been administered (i.e. prolonged seizures);
- History of frequent episodes of serial seizures (i.e. repeated seizures);
- History of convulsive status epilepticus;
- History of first episode requiring emergency dental treatment;
- If there are difficulties monitoring the patient's airway, breathing, circulation, or other vital signs.

In this question, the most likely scenario necessitating summoning emergency help is a history of more than three episodes of jerking movements of the limb in 1 hour; this implies the patient has a history of experiencing repeated seizures.

Further reading

Jevon P. Updated posters to help manage medical emergencies in the dental practice. *Br Dent J*, 2015;219(5):227.

60. A

There are specific conditions that would require calling 999 and transfer to hospital for each medical emergency—they are as follows:

- Asthma:
  - ◆ No response to initial management
  - ◆ Patient has signs of severe and life threating asthma (i.e. tachycardia, cyanosed, distressed, exhaustion, and decreased consciousness levels)
  - ◆ Patient requiring additional doses of bronchodilator (salbutamol)
- Anaphylaxis:
  - ◆ No response to initial management
  - ◆ All patients treated for an anaphylactic reaction should be sent to hospital by ambulance for further assessment, irrespective of any initial recovery
- Epileptic seizure:
  - ◆ No response to initial management
  - ◆ Repeated and atypical seizures
  - ◆ If injury occurs
  - ◆ Status epilepticus
  - ◆ High risk of recurrence
  - ◆ First episode
  - ◆ Difficulty monitoring the individual's condition
- Hypoglycaemia:
  - ◆ No response to initial management
  - ◆ Difficulty during management
- Syncope:
  - ◆ No response to initial management (most likely not syncope)

The most plausible option is an anaphylactic attack.

Rationale: Because patients can develop a second anaphylactic response several hours later in response to the initial allergen exposure, all patients treated for an anaphylactic reaction should be sent to hospital by ambulance for further assessment, irrespective of any initial recovery.

This second phase also known as a biphasic reaction, which usually occurs after an asymptomatic period of up to 72 hours, but most occur within 8 hours after the initial reaction. Therefore, patients MUST be observed for at least 6 hours after the initial symptoms of anaphylaxis subside, and maybe for 12 hours if considered appropriate. This is best carried out in a hospital setting.

Further reading

Jevon P. Updated posters to help manage medical emergencies in the dental practice. *Br Dent J*, 2015;219(5):227.

Rheumatological diseases

61. D

All of the options with exception of trigeminal neuralgia are inflammatory disorders.

Polymyalgia rheumatica, giant cell arteritis, and Takayasu's arteritis are vascultic conditions. Polymyositis is an inflammatory myopathy. Trigeminal neuralgia is a condition of neuropathic facial pain.

Polymyalgia rheumatica—characterized by a prominent systemic inflammatory response with undetectable inflammation of blood vessels; occurs in people >50 years.

Clinical features—severe stiffness and pain in the girdle muscles (i.e. neck, shoulders, buttocks, and thighs); the forearms, hands, calves, and feet usually are not affected. Symptoms of systemic inflammation (e.g. anorexia, depression, fever, malaise, night sweats, weight loss). Shoulder pain is the most common symptom.

Investigation findings—mild, normochromic, normocytic anaemia, ESR greater than 50 mm per hour.

Consequences—the pain and stiffness experienced in the shoulders and upper arms can cause significant disability thus make hygiene and self-care tasks difficult.

Giant cell arteritis (GCA) (temporal arteritis)—syndrome of systemic inflammation accompanied by vascular manifestations. Inflammation of the artery may cause narrowing or occlusion of the blood vessel leading to ischaemia distal to the lesion. GCA most commonly affects branches of the internal and external carotid arteries particularly the temporal artery. Occur in people age 50 years or older.

Clinical features—headaches, jaw claudication, scalp tenderness visual symptoms (diplopia, visual field cuts, partially obscured vision), constitutional symptoms include fever, weight loss, malaise, depression.

Investigation findings—anaemia, ESR greater than 50 mm per hour, abnormal temporal artery on biopsy.

Consequences—can lead to blindness, if not diagnosed and treated in a timely manner.

Takayasu' arteritis—is a chronic inflammatory arteritis affecting large vessels, predominantly the aorta and its main branches. It is a rare disease and presents in the second and third decade of life.

Clinical features—non-specific features include fever, night sweats, malaise, weight loss, arthralgia, myalgia, and mild anaemia. Diminished or absent pulses associated with limb claudication and blood pressure discrepancies, vascular bruits, hypertension, Takayasu retinopathy.

Investigations—angiography is the gold standard, Raised ESR.

Complications—dissection and rupture of the blood vessels.

Polymyositis—rare autoimmune disease characterized by proximal skeletal muscle weakness, raised muscle enzymes (creatinine kinase), and extramuscular involvement (e.g. lungs resulting in interstitial lung disease).

Clinical features—symmetrical, bilateral, proximal muscle weakness manifesting as difficulty in combing hair or reaching for objects above their head with upper limb muscle involvement. Lower limb involvement typically presents with difficulty standing up from a chair or walking up stairs.

Investigation findings—raised creatinine kinase up to 50 times above normal limits, characteristic findings on muscle biopsy is the gold standard for diagnosis; MRI imaging and electromyography are also useful modalities for guiding treatment.

When all of the following variables are taken into consideration, the most plausible option is temporal (giant cell) arteritis for the following reasons:

- Age of onset >50 year excludes Takayasu's arteritis which occurs before 40 years. The onset of the disease has been reported as the single most discriminatory factor between GCA and Takayasu's arteritis. GCA and polymyositis rheumatica are rare in patients younger than 50 years.
- The presence of jaw claudication, scalp tenderness, and pain excludes polymyositis rheumatica which is associated with pain and aches in the shoulder and limb muscles alongside non-specific prodromal features.
- A high ESR >50 mm per hour includes GCA and polymyositis rheumatic but excludes polymyositis associated with raised creatinine kinase and trigeminal neuralgia.
- Site of involvement—Takayasu's is also excluded as it affects large blood vessels (i.e. aorta and its main branches). In contrast GCA has a predilection for small to medium sized blood vessels with the branches of the internal and external carotid arteries notably the temporal artery being the site of predilection. Note, aortic involvement is reported in 10–15% of patients with GCA. No detectable vascular involvement is seen in polymyositis rheumatica.
- The absence of unilateral orofacial pain within the facial or intraoral trigeminal territory and paroxysmal character of pain. The absence of pain triggered by typical manoeuvres also excludes trigeminal neuralgia.

GCA is treated with high dose of prednisone (usually 40–60 mg per day). In patients with visual symptoms, treatment often is initiated with intravenous formulations, such as methylprednisolone. Note treatment should not be delayed while awaiting temporal artery biopsy as this has no effect on biopsy results for up to 4 weeks after commencing management.

Further reading

Unwin B, Williams CM, Gilliland W. Polymyalgia rheumatica and giant cell arteritis. *Am Fam Physician*, 2006;74(9):1547–54.

62. D

Paget's disease of bone is characterized by focal areas of increased and disorganized bone remodelling affecting one or more bones throughout the skeleton. The axial skeleton, most frequently affecting the pelvis, femur, lumbar spine, skull, and tibia are preferential targets. Paget's disease is rare before the age of 55 years. It may present as an incidental finding on radiographic examination or biochemical testing, i.e. an abnormal radiograph or elevated serum alkaline phosphatase level, respectively, in a patient whose health is being investigated for other reasons. For other patients, bone pain is the reason for seeking medical attention.

Complications of Paget's disease include bone pain due to osteoarthritis, spinal stenosis, or pseudo fracture, deafness in patients with skull involvement, osteosarcoma, high output cardiac failure, and obstructive hydrocephalus (which is rare).

Nitrogen-containing bisphosphonates (amino bisphosphonates) such as alendronate, pamidronate, risedronate, and zoledronic acid are the drugs of first choice in the treatment of Paget's disease of bone. They preferentially target affected sites and are highly effective at suppressing the increased bone turnover and stabilizing structural changes.

Bone pain and muscle pain are possible complications associated with infusion of intravenous bisphosphonates. This usually occurs with 1–3 days after the infusion (acute phase response) and subsides with 7 days without treatment. Hearing loss and osteosarcoma are possible complications of the disease. However ongoing treatment with intravenous bisphosphonates reduces the likelihood of developing these complications. A side effect that dentists are usually concerned about in patients treated with intravenous bisphosphonates is medication-related osteonecrosis of the jaw (MRONJ). Therefore, osteonecrosis is the most plausible option.

Further reading

American Association of Oral and Maxillofacial Surgeons. *Medication-Related Osteonecrosis of the Jaw—2014 Update.* Available at: https://www.aaoms.org/images/uploads/pdfs/mronj_position_paper.pdf

Ralston SH. Paget's disease of bone. *N Engl J Med*, 2013;368(7):644–50.

63. E

Graft-versus-host disease (GVHD) is a syndrome in which immunocompetent donor cells recognize and attack host tissues in an immunocompromised recipient. It is a complication of haematopoietic stem cell transplant and can affect many organ systems, including the gastrointestinal tract, liver, skin, mucosa, and lungs. Corticosteroids either alone or in combination with other agents for example cyclosporine, azathioprine, etc. remains the mainstay first-line treatment for GVHD. Prolonged corticosteroid treatment increases risks of developing well documented side effects including immunosuppression resulting in opportunistic fungal and viral infections. Acyclovir was coprescribed as an anti-infective prophylaxis to manage opportunistic viral infections. Other side effects include hyperglycaemia (raised Hb_{A1c}), peptic ulcer disease, osteoporosis, hypertension, cataracts, depression, weight gain, etc.

Secondary osteoporosis is the most notable side effect of prolonged corticosteroid use in relation to the patient's back pain. It manifests as decreased density of mineralized bone which impairs the mechanical strength of bone thus making them vulnerable to fracture. In osteoporosis, as in hypertension, there is often a long latent period before clinical symptoms or complications develop. Pathologic fractures are the most obvious clinical manifestations of osteoporosis and often can present as an episode of acute back pain. The pain can be described as one which intensifies with sitting or standing and relieved by bed rest in the fully recumbent position. Radiographic changes occur in the axial skeleton and can be assessed by evaluation of BMD. Serum calcium and phosphate levels are typically normal.

Osteomalacia refers to inadequately mineralized bone matrix, bone density is usually normal. In children, osteomalacia is recognized as rickets. Causes of osteomalacia include chronic renal failure, malabsorption, vitamin D deficiency, vitamin D pathway abnormalities, and hypophosphataemic syndromes. Osteomalacia can present clinically as generalized bone pain, tenderness, and generalized myopathy. Radiographic changes are seen in appendicular skeleton. Serum calcium and phosphate levels are chronically low with raised alkaline phosphatase.

Osteoarthritis is a degenerative joint disease in adults characterized by progressive loss and destruction of articular cartilage, thickening of the subchondral bone, formation of osteophytes, variable degrees of inflammation of the synovium, degeneration of ligaments, and menisci of the knee and hypertrophy of the joint capsule. It primarily affects the elderly. The aetiology of osteoarthritis is multifactorial and includes joint injury, obesity, ageing, and heredity.

Osteomyelitis refers to inflammation of bone and can be categorized as acute and chronic based on pathological findings. Acute osteomyelitis is typically associated with inflammatory bone changes caused by pathogenic bacteria. The symptoms present with two weeks of infection. In chronic osteomyelitis, a sequestrum is present on imaging and it may take up to 6 weeks to become symptomatic after onset of infection.

Osteodystrophy also known as metabolic bone disease is a common complication of chronic kidney disease. The disease is asymptomatic with symptoms only appearing late in its course. The symptoms are non-specific and include pain and stiffness in joints, spontaneous tendon rupture, predisposition to fracture, and proximal muscle weakness. The bone changes seen in osteodystrophy result from a combination of one or the following abnormalities of calcium, phosphorus, parathyroid hormone (PTH), and vitamin D metabolism and abnormalities of bone turnover, mineralization, volume, linear growth, and strength.

Osteoporosis and osteomalacia are the two most plausible options. However, the most likely cause for this patient's back pain considering their long-term use of corticosteroids is osteoporosis. This patient will benefit from bone densitometry, radiographic imaging, and the institution of preventive measures and medical interventions to manage her back pain.

Further reading

Garnett C, Apperley JF, Pavlů J. Treatment and management of graft-versus-host disease: improving response and survival. *Ther Adv Haematol*, 2013;4(6):366–78.

Glaser DL, Kaplan FS. Osteoporosis: definition and clinical presentation. *Spine*, 1997;22(24):12S–16S.

64. E

Diseases that can cause raised bone-derived alkaline phosphatase include Paget's disease, osteosarcoma, metastatic bone disease, for example, metastasis from prostatic cancer, osteomalacia, vitamin D deficiency, rickets, primary hyperthyroidism, renal osteodystrophy from secondary hyperthyroidism.

Acromegaly is caused by an excessive production of growth hormone from the anterior pituitary gland, resulting in excessive growth of body tissues and other metabolic dysfunctions. Patients have characteristic facial features of a large lower jaw, prominent forehead, and large hands and feet. They can also present maxillary widening which can contribute to ill-fitting of a recently fabricated denture. Bone-derived alkaline phosphatase, serum calcium, phosphate, and 25-hydroxyvitamin D are likely to be normal. An oral glucose tolerance test and levels of insulin-like growth factor are diagnostic tests for acromegaly.

Osteomalacia also called adult rickets, rickets, and vitamin D deficiency can cause a moderate rise in alkaline phosphatase levels. Calcium, phosphate, and 25-hydroxyvitamin D are usually abnormal in majority of cases, therefore also not a plausible option.

Osteoporosis is a skeletal condition characterized by decreased density of normally mineralized bone. In asymptomatic osteoporosis, serum levels of calcium, phosphate, and alkaline phosphatase are normal. Alkaline phosphatase levels may rise transiently after a fracture in severe osteoporosis.

Osteosarcoma is a primary mesenchymal tumour that is characterized histologically by the production of osteoid by malignant cells. It is a relatively rare malignancy and can complicate Paget's disease. Clinical features include localized pain and swelling of the affected area. A pathologic fracture may be the presenting sign. Laboratory values are of little utility in osteosarcoma with the exception of alkaline phosphatase and lactate dehydrogenase which offer prognostic information, with an extreme elevation portending a poor outcome.

Paget's disease is a chronic disorder, characterized by focal areas of excessive osteoclastic bone resorption accompanied by a secondary increase in osteoblastic bone formation. Most cases are asymptomatic and are usually incidental findings on image or biochemical evaluation. Clinical features include bone pain, deformity (bowing of tibia or femur), arthropathy, bone fracture, and neurological complications. The most common neurological complication is deafness arising from involvement of the petrous temporal bone. It may be conductive in nature (from involvement of the middle-ear ossicles), sensorineural (from auditory nerve compression or cochlear involvement) or mixed. Other neurological syndromes are uncommon, but include vertigo, spinal cord compression, local compression syndromes, such as cranial nerve palsies, and, rarely, hydrocephalus or brainstem compression from basilar invagination. Skull enlargement is also a complication, involvement of facial or maxillary bones, mandibular parts of the skeleton can contribute to difficulty with wearing new dental prosthesis.

Typically, patients with Paget's disease of bone present with an markedly elevated bone derived alkaline phosphatase level, with otherwise normal levels of calcium, albumin, alkaline phosphatase, and 25-hydroxyvitamin D. 25-hydroxyvitamin D levels may be reduced, this probably reflects the fact that Paget's disease of bone predominantly affects older people, among whom vitamin D deficiency is prevalent.

In conclusion, Paget's disease of bone is the most likely cause of the patient's hearing loss, difficulty with wearing a recently fabricated denture, and markedly raised bone-derived alkaline phosphatase.

Further reading

Walsh JP. Paget's disease of bone. *Med J Aust*, 2004;181(5):262–5.

65. D

Acromegaly (enlargement (*megaly*) of the extremities (*acral*)) is a slowly progressive disease resulting from the increased release of growth hormone (GH) and, consequently, insulin-like growth factor I. In the majority of cases this is induced by a growth hormone-secreting pituitary tumour and more rarely by pituitary hyperplasia or ectopic secretion of GH or GH-releasing hormone. Clinical features include wide hands and feet; broad, stubby fingers and toes; and thickened soft tissues. Characteristic facial appearance includes a rectangular face, an enlarged widened nose, prominent cheekbones, a bulging forehead, thickened lips, and marked wrinkling of the skin. There is a tendency for prognathism, maxillary widening, teeth separation, and jaw malocclusion. Patient may also present comorbidities such as diabetes or glucose intolerance, hypertension, OSAS, cardiomyopathy (mainly left ventricular hypertrophy) and goitre.

Clinical investigations:

Serum insulin-like growth factor 1 measurement requires only one blood sample which can obtained at any time of the day. It is the first-line diagnostic test for this reason.

Serum GH measurement requires more than one sample which must be obtained at a particular time of day (in the morning) to measure basal levels. Due to high growth hormone levels in normal individuals owing to the episodic nature of physiologic growth hormone secretion and the many peaks of GH levels approximately a dozen peaks per day, mainly during sleep, random sampling of serum growth hormone levels can therefore be unreliable.

The prevalence of diabetes and glucose intolerance in patients with acromegaly means serum glucose levels which is typically raised is non-diagnostic.

Parathyroid hyperactivity secondary to acromegaly will cause serum calcium and phosphate levels to be raised hence not diagnostic.

Therefore, the most reliable marker for establishing a diagnosis of acromegaly is the measurement serum insulin-like growth factor 1, the reason being its level in blood is stable throughout the day. In patients with elevated IGF-1, it is recommended that the diagnosis is confirmed by observing a lack of suppression of GH levels (to <1 µg/l) following confirmed hyperglycaemia during an OGTT.

Further reading

Colao A, et al. Acromegaly. *Nat Rev Dis Primers*, 2019;5(1):20.

66. A

Older patients living in care homes are three times more likely to fall than older people living in their own homes. The resultant effect is 10 times more hip fractures in care homes than in other environments. Factors associated with this include physical frailty, long-term medical conditions, physical inactivity, polypharmacy, and unfamiliarity with the environment. Other individual factors include previous falls, being less physically active, cognitive problems such as memory loss, dizziness spells, etc. Factors relating to the environment can also be contributory; examples include poor lighting; wet, slippery, or uneven floors; clutter; inappropriate or unsafe walking aids; loose-fitting footwear, and clothing, etc. Specific conditions acute or temporary medical conditions can also increase the risk of falling due to the effects of their mental and physical health. These conditions include constipation, acute infection including urinary tract infection, chest infections, or pneumonia. Others include dehydration, delirium (sudden severe confusion and rapid changes in brain function associated with mental or physical illness). *Note*: all the factors in the options can contribute to a fall in elderly patients, how the acute onset of the patient symptoms and the associated confusion makes delirium the most plausible option.

Further reading

Care Inspectorate. *Managing Falls and Fractures in Care Homes for Older People, Good Practice Self-Assessment Resource.* Available at: https://www.careinspectorate.com/images/documents/2737/2016/Falls-and-fractures-new-resource-low-res.pdf

National Institute for Health and Care Excellence. Older people in care homes. Local government briefing [LGB25]. Available at: https://www.nice.org.uk/guidance/older) people in care homes pdf

67. D

Osteoporosis is a skeletal condition characterized by decreased density of normally mineralized bone with an increased risk of fracture. Two forms exist: type I presents with accelerated bone loss secondary to oestrogen deficiency which is seen in postmenopausal women; type II is seen in both sexes and is associated with age-related cortical and trabecular bone loss. This typically leads to fractures of the proximal femur in the elderly. Risk factors for osteoporosis include, positive family history, smoking, chronic alcohol abuse, obesity, early menopause, prolonged immobilization, female gender, elderly patient, low dietary calcium and vitamin D, primary hypogonadism, sedentary lifestyle, Caucasian or Asian origin, and chronic disorders such as anorexia nervosa, malabsorption syndromes, Cushing syndrome, chronic renal failure, etc.

In this patient, diet appears to be a significant contributory factor to their osteoporosis and resultant fracture.

Paleo diet: This contains food as natural as possible (i.e. opting for grass-fed meats, abundance of fruits and vegetable, nuts, and seeds). In other words, all versions of a paleo diet encourage lean proteins, fruit, vegetables, and healthy fats from whole foods such as nuts, seeds and olive oil, and grass-fed meat.

Macrobiotic diet: This constitutes well-chewed whole cereal grains (e.g. brown rice, quinoa, rey, teff, millet, and barley). Other constituents include vegetables, beans and legumes, sea vegetables, miso soup, and fish and seafoods, which can be eaten occasionally.

Vegan diet: This contains only plants such as vegetables, grains, nuts, and fruits. Vegans do not eat foods that come from animals, including dairy products and eggs.

Gluten-free diet: This aims to avoid food that contains gluten. Foods rich in calcium and fat-soluble vitamins, for example, meat, fish, potatoes, fruits, and vegetables lentils are naturally gluten-free and can be eaten.

Vegetarian diet: This is rich in grains, pulses, nuts, seeds, vegetables, and fruits with some also choosing to include dairy products including cheese (made using vegetable rennet) and eggs.

The vegan diet is most likely to be associated with development of osteoporosis and an increased risk of fracture because of a deficiency of fat-soluble vitamins (vitamin D), calcium, and other minerals found in fish, red meat, liver, egg yolks, required for development of healthy bones and teeth.

Further reading

BBC Good Food. Available at:https://www.bbcgoodfood.com

NHS. *Prevention: Osteoporosis.* Available at: https://www.nhs.uk/conditions/osteoporosis/pages/prevention.aspx

68. B

See question 61 in the rheumatological disease section for details on polymyalgia rheumatic and Takayasu's arteritis.

Fibromyalgia is a complex syndrome characterized by chronic diffuse or multifocal muscle pain, increased sensitivity to pain aggravated by touching and relived by rest and topical heat, physical exhaustion, and muscle stiffness.

Physical examination is typically unremarkable.

Investigation findings—Laboratory investigations are not useful for establishing a diagnosis.

Polyarteritis nodosa is a systemic necrotizing vasculitis that predominantly targets medium sized arteries and occasionally small sized blood vessels. There are two types, idiopathic and hepatitis B virus associated. Average age of onset is 50 years and older.

Clinical features—are dependent on the organ involved or if there is multiorgan involvement. The disease causes occlusion and rupture of the inflamed arteries thereby causing tissue ischaemia or haemorrhage. The peripheral nervous system and the skin are the most frequently involved. The main neurological manifestation is mononeuritis multiplex, which presents with wrist or foot drop. Cutaneous features, including purpura, livedoid lesions, subcutaneous nodules, and necrotic ulcers. Non-specific constitutional symptom like weight loss, malaise, fever, arthralgia, and myalgia are described. An ontological manifestation of polyarteritis nodosa is hearing loss, which is most often sensorineural. The hearing loss is typically bilateral and of sudden onset.

Investigation findings—Requires the integration of clinical, angiographic, and biopsy findings.

Antineutrophil cytoplasmic antibodies (ANCA) are typically negative excluding other systemic vasculitis, e.g. Churg–Strauss and granulomatosis with polyangiitis (Wegner's granulomatosis).

Treatment—Cyclophosphamide and immunosuppressive agents such as azathioprine and methotrexate are the mainstay for treatment.

GCA (temporal arteritis) is a syndrome of systemic inflammation accompanied by vascular manifestations. Inflammation of the artery may cause narrowing or occlusion of the blood vessel leading to ischaemia distal to the lesion. GCA most commonly affects branches of the internal and external carotid arteries particularly the temporal artery. Occurs in people age 50 years or older.

Clinical features—Headaches, jaw claudication, scalp tenderness visual symptoms (diplopia, visual field cuts, partially obscured vision), constitutional symptoms include fever, weight loss, malaise, depression.

Investigation findings—Anaemia, raised CRP, ESR greater than 50 mm per hour, abnormal temporal artery on biopsy.

Consequences—Can lead to blindness, if not diagnosed and treated in a timely manner.

GCA is treated with high dose of prednisone (usually 40–60 mg per day). In patients with visual symptoms, treatment often is initiated with intravenous formulations, such as methylprednisolone. Note treatment should not be delayed while awaiting temporal artery biopsy as this has no effect on biopsy results for up to four weeks after commencing management.

The clinical scenario closely matches the description of GCA; therefore it is the most plausible option.

Further reading

Unwin B, Williams CM, Gilliland W. Polymyalgia rheumatica and giant cell arteritis. *Am Family Physician*, 2006;74(9):1547–54.

Cardiac diseases

69. A

AF is characterized by a variable R-R interval and fibrillatory waves in lead II and V. Clinical features include palpitations, irregular pulse, cardiac failure and embolic phenomena (chronic AF patient have a six fold increase in developing a stroke). Treatment is aimed at restoring sinus rhythm by correcting the underlying cause, slowing the ventricular rate with atrioventricular (AV) blocking drugs and anticoagulation to prevent thromboembolic complications.

Atrial flutter often caused by a single re-entrant circuit in the right atrium is characterized by atrial rate between 250 and 300 bpm. The ECG trace shows a sawtooth pattern in lead II and III. Atrial embolism is rare in atrial flutter because of the presence of a discrete atrial mechanical systole after each electrical flutter, hence the risk of an embolic phenomena is negligible. Atrioventricular regurgitation also does not occur in atrial flutter. Cardioversion with low voltage direct current shock is the treatment of choice. To maintain sinus rhythm, an antiarrhythmic drug (verapamil, amiodarone, procainamide) may be prescribed following cardioversion.

Bradycardia is characterized by regular heart rates slower than 60 bpm. A few of the many aetiological factors include sick sinus syndrome, physiological, particularly in athletes and drugs induced with beta blockers and calcium channel blockers, underlying medical conditions (e.g. hypothyroidism, infections, acute myocardial infarction vagal stimulation, etc.). Treatment is aimed at correcting the underlying cause if medication induced, consider withdrawing medication, or where medication is an absolute requirement, a permanent pacemaker may be considered. If caused by infection or underlying thyroid abnormality, the patient should be appropriately managed.

Sinus tachycardia is characterized by regular heart rates of between 100 and 160 bpm. There are a variety of aetiologies including thyrotoxicosis, anxiety, phaeochromocytoma, tetanus, fever, sympathomimetic stimulation or drug effect, shock, pain, etc. Treatment should be aimed at correcting the underlying cause (i.e. treat underlying fever, thyroid or adrenal abnormalities, etc.). Beta blockers may be required if inappropriate sympathetic hyperactivity (phaeochromocytoma or thyrotoxic crisis) is the underlying cause of the tachycardia.

Ventricular tachycardia is characterized by three or more consecutive ectopic ventricular pulse having the same contour and separated by a fixed interval. The rate ranges between 130 and 180 bpm. In most cases, the R–R intervals are regular and the QRS complexes are usually uniform and monomorphic. Clinical features include features of hypotension, shock, angina, or cardiac failure due to the underlying myocardial disease. Treatment involves cardioversion followed by rate controlling drugs (e.g. beta blockers, amiodarone, etc.).

AF is the most likely cardiac arrhythmia this patient is being managed for, as the medications used closely matches the treatment aims (i.e. rivaroxaban, a novel oral anticoagulant) to manage the risk of thromboembolic complications, warfarin can also achieve this treatment aim. Atenolol, a beta-adrenergic receptor blocker, for rate control (to reduce the ventricular rate). Amiodarone which prolongs action potential is used for rate control (in this case reduce the ventricular rate) and to restore sinus rhythm. Simvastatin, a statin, used to manage hypercholesterolaemia, a risk factor for cardiovascular disease.

Further reading

Durham D, Worthley LI. Cardiac arrhythmias: diagnosis and management: the tachycardias. *Crit Care Resusc*, 2002;4(1):35.

Greenwood M, Meechan JG. General medicine and surgery for dental practitioners part 1: cardiovascular system. *Br Dent J*, 2003;194(10): 537–42.

70. A

Losartan, a benzyl-substituted imidazole, is a specific competitive antagonist of angiotensin II receptor subtype 1 (AT_1) it blocks angiotensin II from binding to AT_1 and AT_2 receptors. AT_1-receptor mediates all the classical effects of angiotensin II (i.e. vasoconstriction, aldosterone release, sympathetic activation, and other potentially harmful effects on the cardiovascular system while the functional role of AT_2 is unclear). In other words, blockade of the AT_1 receptor causes a reduction in blood pressure by blocking vasoconstriction and resulting in vasodilation. Other examples of angiotensin II receptor antagonists are irbesartan, telmisartan, etc.

Some examples of the other classes of antihypertensive drugs in the options are as follows:

- Angiotensin-converting enzyme inhibitors—enalapril, ramipril, lisinopril, captopril, trandolapril
- β adrenergic receptor blockers—atenolol, bisoprolol, sotalol, labetalol, nadolol
- Loop diuretic—furosemide, bumetanide, torsemide
- Thiazide—bendroflumethiazide, hydrochlorothiazide, indapamide

Further reading

National Institute for Health and Care Excellence. *BNF*. Available at: https://bnf.nice.org.uk/

Oliverio MI, Coffman TM. Angiotensin-II receptors: new targets for antihypertensive therapy. *Clin Cardiol*, 1997;20(1):3–6.

71. B

Corneal arcus refers to a grey-white or yellowish opacity located near the periphery of the cornea but separated from the limbic margin by a clear corneal zone called the lucid interval of Vogt.

The yellowish lesions at the inner canthus of the eye and on the eyelids are referred to xanthelasma.

Angina is a manifestation of atherosclerotic cardiovascular disease.

All three features are indicative of hyperlipidaemia but may be seen in normolipidemic patients.

Causes of hypercholesterolaemia:

- Primary hypercholesterolaemia—Familial hypercholesterolaemia
- Secondary hypercholesterolaemia—Hypothyroidism, nephrotic syndrome, Cushing's syndrome, obstructive jaundice, anorexia nervosa, thiazide diuretics, ciclosporin, etc.

The development of corneal arcus, tendon xanthomas, and cutaneous xanthelasmas and atherosclerotic cardiovascular disease, are related to the extent (serum level) and duration (age) of the elevated LDL levels. In other words, there is a higher frequency of developing these features in familial hypercholesterolaemia characterized by marked elevations in LDL levels from birth compared to secondary hypercholesterolaemia. Hence, patients with familial hypercholesterolaemia develop these features at a younger age (before 50 years).

Nephrotic syndrome, Cushing's syndrome, obstructive jaundice, and hypothyroidism are all not plausible because they are secondary causes of hypercholesterolaemia. While patients with secondary hypercholesterolaemia can also develop bilateral corneal arcus, atherosclerotic cardiovascular disease (angina) and cutaneous xanthelasma, it tends to occur at a much older age. Considering the patient is young (29 years old), the most likely cause of their bilateral corneal arcus, atherosclerotic cardiovascular disease (angina), and cutaneous xanthelasma is familial hypercholesterolaemia. Corneal arcus has been reported in patients as young as 13 years of age in the presence of severe familial hypercholesterolemia.

Further reading

Bhatnagar D, Soran H, Durrington PN. Hypercholesterolaemia and its management. *BMJ*, 2008;337:a993.

Fernández A, Sorokin A, Thompson PD. Corneal arcus as coronary artery disease risk factor. *Atherosclerosis*, 2007;193(2):235–40.

72. E

Indapamide is a thiazide diuretic; other examples include hydrochlorothiazide, bendroflumethiazide.

Bisoprolol is a β adrenergic receptor blocker, other examples include atenolol, sotalol, labetalol, nadolol.

α adrenergic receptor blocker—doxazosin, tamsulosin, alfuzosin, prazosin, terazosin.

Potassium channel blockers—dofetilide, ibutilide.

Amlodipine is a calcium channel blocker; other examples include nifedipine, verapamil.

Aldosterone antagonist—spironolactone, eplerenone.

Osmotic diuretic—mannitol.

Potassium sparing diuretics—amiloride hydrochloride and triamterene.

Loop diuretic—furosemide, bumetanide, torsemide.

Indapamide, bisoprolol and amlodipine are thiazide diuretic, β adrenergic receptor blocker and calcium channel blocker, respectively. They are used to manage the patient's hypertension.

Further reading

National Institute for Health and Care Excellence. *BNF*. Available at: https://bnf.nice.org.uk/

73. C

Ventricular fibrillation (VF) and pulseless ventricular tachycardia (VT) are primary arrhythmic events that can cause out-of-hospital cardiac arrest. Both are shockable rhythms therefore managed by delivering electrical shocks with an AED together with effective cardiopulmonary resuscitation (CPR).

VT shows as a wide, regular, and very rapid rhythm on ECG monitor or tracing. It is a poorly perfusing rhythm thus patients may present with a pulse or pulseless. Most patients with VT are unconscious and pulseless. Defibrillation to 'reset' the heart, i.e. make primary pacemaker (usually the sinoatrial node) to start generating impulses is required. These together with effective CPR are crucial for survival.

VF looks like a frenetically disorganized wavy line on ECG tracing or monitor. In VF, the heart quivers ineffectively and no blood is pumped out of the heart. Defibrillation by an AED is required to terminate the rhythm.

Pulseless electrical activity (PEA) and asystole are not amenable to shock hence non-shockable rhythms. They are managed by performing good CPR and arranging urgent transfer to hospital for specialized care.

Supraventricular tachycardia (SVT) as the name implies originates above the ventricles. Patients have a rapid rhythm with a heart rate greater than 150 beats per minute. Patients may be relatively stable with few symptoms, or profoundly unstable with severe signs and symptoms related to the rapid heart rate. Unstable patients or those who do not respond to medication will require synchronized cardioversion, rather than defibrillation.

The most likely arrhythmia detected by the AED which is amenable to defibrillation is pulseless VT.

Further reading

ACLS. *Shockable Rhythms.* Available at: https://acls.com/free-resources/knowledge-base/vf-pvt/shockable-rhythms

Resuscitation Council UK. *Guidelines: Adult Advanced Life Support.* Available at: https://www.resus.org.uk/resuscitation-guidelines/adult-advanced-life-support/#algorithm

74. B

Dabigatran is a novel oral anticoagulants (NOAC) and a direct thrombin inhibitor (prevents the conversion of fibrinogen to fibrin, thereby preventing clot formation). Other NOACs include rivaroxaban apixaban and edoxaban, they are direct factor Xa (FXa) inhibitors (block the conversion of prothrombin into thrombin). All are used as alternatives to vitamin K antagonists (warfarin) to limit the risk of potential stroke and systemic embolism for individuals with non-valvular AF. In comparison to vitamin K antagonists (warfarin), they offer the advantage of more predictable anticoagulant effect, rapid onset and offset of action, no requirement for constant monitoring, and a very low potential for drug–drug interaction allowing for concurrent use of other medications. Furthermore, their absorption is unaffected in the presence of food and there is no need for regular dose adjustments.

As vitamin K is used to reverse warfarin effects, idarucizumab is used for reversal of the anticoagulant effects of dabigatran. This is particularly useful in cases where emergency surgery is needed or patient experiencing life-threatening or uncontrolled bleeding. Antidotes for oral direct FXa inhibitors (rivaroxaban apixaban and edoxaban) are currently being developed as at the time of publication.

Conventional tests such as INR, PT, and partial thromboplastin time (aPTT) are not useful for monitoring the effects of dabigatran.

The patient's surgical extraction of an unerupted third molar would require flap raising, bone removal, and would result in a large postoperative wound. Therefore, the procedure is considered to be high risk for postoperative bleeding complication. Hence, NOAC discontinuation is recommended as a primary measure for preventing a bleeding complication. Local haemostatic measures and suturing to close the resultant wound are reactive/secondary measures that can be utilized if the need arises after the procedure.

For dabigatran, discontinue 24–48 hours prior to surgery and recommence administration postoperatively following haemostasis. Since dabigatran is taken twice daily, a more patient friendly instruction would be to miss their morning dose and take their evening dose at the usual time as long as it is no longer than 4 hours after haemostasis has been achieved.

For rivaroxaban taken once daily, interruption at 24 hours prior to the dental procedure is recommended. In other words, if taken routinely in the morning, do not take on the morning of the extraction and recommence 4 hours after haemostasis has been achieved. If taken in the evening, they can take this at the usual time of day as long as no earlier than 4 hours after haemostasis has been achieved.

In conclusion, while options B and C are both appropriate precautions to be taken in managing this patient, option B is the most appropriate, therefore the most plausible option.

Further reading

Fortier K, Shroff D, Reebye UN. An overview and analysis of novel oral anticoagulants and their dental implications. *Gerodontology,* 2018;35(2):78–86.

SDCEP. [Dental clinical guidance] *Scottish Dental Clinical Effectiveness Programme,* August 2015. Available at: http://www.sdcep.org.uk/

Neurological diseases

75. D

Cranial nerve III—oculomotor nerve is a motor nerve and supplies the inferior oblique, superior, inferior, and medial rectus and palpebrae superioris. It also supplies the pupillary sphincter

Cranial nerve V—trigeminal nerve is mainly sensory through its three main branches ophthalmic, maxillary, and mandibular and motor to the muscles of mastication.

Cranial nerve VI—abducents nerve is a motor nerve to the lateral rectus muscle.

Cranial nerve VII—facial nerve is a mixed cranial nerve with motor (muscles of facial expression), parasympathetic (salivary glands (submandibular and sublingual) and mucous glands of mouth and nose), sensory branches (part of external ear) and special sensory (anterior two-thirds of tongue via chorda tympani). It originates in the brainstem and travels through the temporal bone before exiting the stylomastoid foramen. The extratemporal branches of the facial nerve are located within the body of the parotid gland and divide it into superficial and deep lobes before innervating the muscles of facial expression via its terminal branches. They include temporal, zygomatic, buccal, mandibular, and cervical branches.

Cranial nerve VIII—vestibulocochlear nerve is sensory nerve responsible for hearing and balance.

Direct infiltration and destruction of the cranial VII nerve by tumour cells from parotid gland malignancies including adenoid cystic carcinoma, squamous cell carcinoma, and salivary duct carcinoma can cause facial nerve paralysis. Up to 33% of patients with malignant parotid gland lesions have facial nerve involvement. Facial nerve paralysis arising from malignant parotid gland lesion is strongly predictive for a shorter disease-free survival.

Further reading

Wierzbicka M, Kopeć T, Szyfter W, Kereiakes T, Bem G. The presence of facial nerve weakness on diagnosis of a parotid gland malignant process. *Eur Arch Otorhino-Laryngol*, 2012;269(4):1177–82.

76. E

Movement of an enlarged thyroid gland on protrusion of the tongue reflects the embryonic origin of the thyroid gland from the foramen caecum at the base of the tongue

An adenomatoid nodule (a single enlarged nodule in the thyroid gland), multinodular goitre (diffuse enlargement of the thyroid with varying degree of nodularity) and a follicular adenoma (a benign encapsulated neoplasm of follicular epithelial origin) are not plausible causes because they are benign lesions. However, if large enough they can compress on the larynx and trachea resulting in difficulty in breathing and stridor.

Papillary thyroid carcinoma is the most common malignant thyroid neoplasm. Patient typically present with a solitary, painless (asymptomatic) neck swelling with or without cervical lymphadenopathy. If large enough they can also cause dysphagia, stridor, and cough by compressing on the larynx and trachea. This is also not a plausible option.

Undifferentiated carcinoma also known as anaplastic carcinoma and pleomorphic carcinoma is a highly aggressive malignant neoplasm composed of undifferentiated thyroid follicular cells. This tumour is typically rapidly enlarging, fixed, and hard neck masses capable of extending into surrounding soft tissues and organs. The widely infiltrative nature of the neoplasm causes hoarseness, dysphagia, difficulty breathing, pain, and vocal cord paralysis. Weight loss and malaise are also suggestive of malignancy.

Therefore, undifferentiated carcinoma which is seen in patient's above 60 years is the most plausible option for the patient's clinical presentation.

Further reading

Thompson LD, Bishop JA. *Head and Neck Pathology E-book: A Volume in the Series: Foundations in Diagnostic Pathology.* London, UK: Elsevier Health Sciences; 2017.

77. A

Herpes zoster (HZ) is a clinical manifestation of the reactivation of latent varicella zoster virus infection. Varicella zoster virus (VZV) usually persists asymptomatically in the dorsal root ganglia of anyone who has had chickenpox. When there is diminished cell mediated immunity (elderly people, patients with lymphoma, those receiving chemotherapy or steroids, and people with HIV), the virus is reactivated from its dormant state. Following reactivation, the virus replicates and travels along the sensory nerve fibres to cause unilateral lesions confined to a dermatome supplied by that nerve (does not cross midline). The cardinal features of HZ are pain and a rash. The pain of the acute phase of HZ is caused by VZV-induced cytopathic damage to nerve cells in the sensory ganglia and in the peripheral sensory nerves during the descent of the reactivated VZV. The rash is typically a vesicular eruption, affects a single dermatome, and lasts for 3–5 days before the lesion pustulates and become crusted. The vesicular rash is thought to be due to the direct cytopathic effect of VZV on epithelial cells.

The most frequent site of reactivation is the thoracic nerves followed by the ophthalmic division of the trigeminal nerve (HZ ophthalmicus), which can progress to involve all structures of the eye. If the mucocutaneous division of the VII cranial nerve, which innervates the ear and side of the tongue is involved, the development of lesions in the ear and facial paralysis are known as Ramsay Hunt syndrome.

HZ ophthalmicus is particularly aggressive and must be treated with antivirals, even if more than 72 hours have elapsed since onset. Oral antiviral agents together with topical antiviral cream applied to the eye and corticosteroids where appropriate. Complications of acute ophthalmic zoster include conjunctivitis, episcleritis, and scleritis, keratitis, iridocyclitis choroiditis, papillitis, oculomotor palsy, retinitis, and optic atrophy.

External auditory canal rash and facial paralysis are features of Ramsay Hunt syndrome and not HZ ophthalmicus. HZ is associated with vesicular and not follicular-type rash. The vesicles show dermatome involvement and usually do not cross the midline. Therefore, the most plausible option which is characteristic of HZ infection its localization to a specific dermatome.

Further reading

Le P, Rothberg M. Herpes zoster infection. *BMJ*, 2019; 364:k5095.

78. D

Convergent squint, an inability to fully abduct the left eye on lateral gaze and a history of diplopia is characteristic of lateral rectus palsy. The lateral rectus muscle is supplied by the abducent nerve, cranial nerve VI. Other cranial nerves which supply extraocular muscles of the eyes are oculomotor (III) and trochlear (IV). CN IV supplies the superior oblique muscle responsible for moving the eyes downwards and medially towards the nose. CN III supplies the inferior oblique (elevates the adducted eye), superior (elevates the eye), medial (adducts the eye) and inferior (depresses the eye) recti muscles as well as the ciliary muscle, the constrictor of the pupil and the muscle that raised the upper eyelid.

CN V and VII, the trigeminal and facial nerve, respectively, do not influence eye movements.

Hint: SO4 LR6 meaning superior oblique supplied by cranial nerve IV (trochlear), lateral rectus supplied by cranial nerve VI (abducent) and the remaining extraocular muscle of the eye including the pupillary sphincter is supplied by cranial nerve III (oculomotor nerve).

Further reading

Scully C. Chapter 13: Neurology. In: Scully C (ed.). *Scully's Medical Problems in Dentistry*, 7th Edition. Edinburgh, UK: Churchill Livingston/Elsevier, 2014.

79. B

CN III is a motor and sensory nerve. Motor to extrinsic muscles of the eye including the inferior oblique (elevates the adducted eye), superior (elevates the eye), medial (adducts the eye), and inferior (depresses the eye) recti muscles. The palpebrae superioris (ciliary muscle) constricts the pupil and pupillary sphincter raises the upper eyelid. Weakness of elevation and adduction (i.e. eye looks down and out on forward gaze associated with ptosis) and a dilated unreactive pupil is indicative of a CN III (oculomotor) nerve lesion. Trauma, multiple sclerosis, diabetes, compression from a neoplasm, compression from an aneurysm, etc., are possible causes of cranial III palsy.

Cranial nerve II (optic) is a sensory nerve and is responsible for vision.

Cranial nerve IV (trigeminal nerve) is sensory via the ophthalmic, maxillary, and mandibular branches. The mandibular branch has a motor component that supplies the muscle of mastication.

Cranial nerve VI (abducent) is pure motor and supplies the lateral rectus muscle only.

Cranial nerve VII (facial) is motor, sensory, and special sensory. Motor to the muscle of facial expression, sensory to part of the skin of the external auditory meatus via the auriculotemporal nerve and special sensory to the anterior two-thirds of the tongue via chorda tympani.

Therefore CNIII (oculomotor) is the most plausible option.

Further reading

Gray D, Toghill PJ. Chapter 7: Basic guide to diseases of the nervous system. In: Gray D, Toghill PJ (eds). *An Introduction to the Symptoms and Signs of Clinical Medicine: A Hands-on Guide to Developing Core Skills*. Taylor & Francis, 2000.

Endocrine diseases

80. C

The clinical features (i.e. bulging eyes, thin patient, excessive sweating, and heat intolerance) are characteristic of hyperthyroidism (increase in thyroid hormone secretion and circulation). The most common cause of hyperthyroidism is Grave's disease, followed by a toxic nodular goitre. Other causes can include factitious ingestion of excess thyroid hormones, thyroiditis, etc. Sinus tachycardia, AF, and atrial flutter can be associated with hyperthyroidism. Sinus tachycardia is associated with increased sympathetic stimulation resulting increased heart between 100 and 160 bpm while AF is characterized by irregular beats, increased heart >100 bpm, palpitations, and embolic phenomena. Atrial flutter is associated with atrial rate between 250 and 300 bpm. In a 2:1 AV block, the ventricular rate will be 150 bpm. Only about 5% of patients with hyperthyroidism can present pure atrial flutter.

VT is associated with heart rate in the range of 130–180 bpm. In contrast to sinus tachycardia, underlying ischaemic heart disease is the most common cause of VT. Other causes include structural heart disease, electrolyte imbalance (hypokalaemia, hypocalcaemia, hypomagnesaemia), drug abuse (cocaine), digitalis toxicity, etc.

VF is associated loss of an orderly sequence of ventricular myocardial contraction caused by a random and chaotic spread of electrical activity. During VF, the heart rate is too high to allow adequate pumping of blood resulting in loss of cardiac output and absence of cerebral perfusion and ultimately death if not treated. Ischaemic heart disease and cardiomyopathies are possible causes.

Both VT and VF are the most common causes of sudden cardiac death.

Sinus bradycardia is associated with regular heart rates slower than 60 bpm. Causes include sick sinus syndrome, physiological particularly in athletes, drugs induced with beta blockers and calcium channel blockers, underlying medical conditions (e.g. hypothyroidism, infections, acute myocardial infarction, vagal stimulation, etc.).

Sinus tachycardia and atrial flutter are both plausible options. However, sinus tachycardia is the most plausible option as it is the more common cardiac arrhythmia in hyperthyroid patients.

Further reading

Jayaprasad N, Francis J. Atrial fibrillation and hyperthyroidism. *Indian Pacing Electrophysiol J*, 2005;5(4):305.

81. D

Table 2.7 Autoimmune diseases and their corresponding autoantigens, autoantibodies, target organs, consequences, and clinical manifestations

Disease	Antigen	Autoantibodies	Target organ	Consequence	Clinical manifestations
Grave's disease	Thyroid-stimulating hormone receptor	Antithyroid-stimulating hormone receptor autoantibodies	Thyroid follicles	Hyperthyroidism	Tachycardia, Heat intolerance, sweating, fatigue, weight loss, palpitations, hypertension, anxiety, eyelid retraction, proptosis
Addison's disease	21 hydroxylase	21 hydroxylase autoantibodies	Adrenal glands	Destruction of adrenal cortex	Weight loss, anorexia, fatigue, nausea and vomiting, abdominal pain, postural hypotension, salt craving, low blood glucose
Pernicious anaemia	Intrinsic factor	Intrinsic factor autoantibodies	Stomach	Destruction of gastric parietal cells	Macrocytic anaemia, glossitis, peripheral neuropathies, memory loss
Myasthenia gravis	Post-synaptic acetyl choline receptor	Acetyl choline autoantibodies	Skeletal muscle	Inhibition of neuromuscular transmission	Muscle weakness, diplopia, ptosis, limb weakness, slurred speech, dysphagia, choking, neck weakness, exertional dyspnoea
Hashimoto's thyroiditis	Thyroglobulin and thyroid microsomes	Thyroglobulin (Tg-Ab) and thyroid peroxidase (TPO-Ab) autoantibodies	Thyroid gland	Destruction of thyroid epithelial cells and fibrosis resulting in hypothyroidism	Constipation, dry, cold yellowish and thickened skin, bradycardia, depression, inability to concentrate, memory loss, weight gain, lassitude, hair loss, menstrual disturbance

Table 2.7 summarizes the key features of the autoimmune conditions associated with each autoantibody in the options. The patient's clinical manifestations as observed by their GDP (i.e. hair loss, fatigue, and lassitude, depression, weight gain, periorbital puffiness) are most in keeping with hypothyroidism. Hashimoto's thyroiditis is an autoimmune disease associated with circulating autoantibodies to thyroglobulin (Tg-Ab) and thyroperioxidase (TPO-Ab). These autoantibodies attack the thyroid gland and impair their ability to produce thyroid hormones resulting in a hypothyroid state. Hashimoto's thyroiditis is considered the most common cause of hypothyroidism.

Note that the autoantibody to TSH receptor causes Grave's disease. The antibody simulates the action of TSH, thereby inducing thyroid hormone synthesis and thyroid gland growth and causing hyperthyroidism. For this reason, it is not a plausible option.

Further reading

Caturegli P, De Remigis A, Rose NR. Hashimoto thyroiditis: clinical and diagnostic criteria. *Autoimmun Rev*, 2014;13(4–5):391–7.

82. A

AD (also known as primary adrenal insufficiency) is a chronic disorder of the adrenal cortex resulting in inadequate secretion of glucocorticoid and mineralocorticoid. Causes of AD include autoimmune adrenalitis in the Western world, infectious disease such as tuberculosis, fungal infections (histoplasmosis, Cryptococcus) and cytomegalovirus in the developing world. Acute haemorrhage in meningococcal septicaemia is also a cause. Clinical features include weakness, fatigue, weight loss, abdominal pain, anorexia, low blood glucose, low blood pressure, postural hypotension, and salt craving. Primary adrenal insufficiency causes an activation of the pituitary gland leading to an increased release of adrenocorticotropin (ACTH) and melanocyte-stimulating hormone (MSH) as part of a negative feedback mechanism. Hypersecretion of ACTH and other pro-opiomelanocortin derived peptides stimulate melanocytes in the skin and mucosa *via* MSH receptor inducing skin and oral mucosa pigmentation. In the oral cavity, this can manifest as bilateral hyperpigmentation involving the buccal mucosa, gingiva, vermillion border of the lower lip or alveolar mucosa.

PJS is an autosomal-dominant disorder characterized by hamartomatous gastrointestinal polyposis and melanin pigmentation of the skin and mucous membranes. The polyps occur throughout the whole digestive tract with a predilection for the small bowel where they typically cause recurrent intussusceptions or intestinal obstruction. Pigmentation of skin and mucous membranes presents as irregularly distributed light to dark brownish macules of 1–5 mm diameter. Within the oral cavity, the vermillion border of the lips, buccal mucosa, gums, and hard palate are common sites of presentation. Smaller and darker skin macules can also be found around the mouth, nose, and eyes. Chronic or recurrent blood loss from gastrointestinal tract can cause iron deficiency anaemia.

Conn's syndrome is caused by a tumour in the zona glomerulosa of the adrenal gland causing excessive production of aldosterone. The clinical picture is that of hypertension with sequalae of headache, polyuria, and polydipsia. Muscle weakness and spasm due to hypokalaemia is also a consequence.

Cowden disease is a multisystem disorder involving increased risks for a number of malignancies as well as benign hamartomatous overgrowth of various tissues. Manifestations of Cowden syndrome include mucocutaneous lesions (trichilemmomas, acral keratosis, papillomatous nodules), thyroid abnormalities (goitre, adenoma, papillary thyroid cancer), breast lesion (fibrocystic disease/fibroadenoma, adenocarcinoma), gastrointestinal tract (hamartomatous polyps), uterine leiomyoma, etc.

Cushing's syndrome—there is pathologic hypercortisolism as a result of excessive ACTH production, or autonomous adrenal production of cortisol. It is associated with significant comorbidities, including hypertension, diabetes, coagulopathy, cardiovascular disease, infections, and fractures. Clinical features include weight gain, fatigue, growth retardation in children, insomnia, on the skin; thin skin, easy bruising, poor wound healing, striae, hirsutism, acne, moon face, mucocutaneous hyperpigmentation, redistribution of adipose tissue (buffalo hump), and accentuation of previous personality/psychiatric disorder.

Conn's syndrome and Cushing's syndrome are associated with hypertension, therefore not plausible options. From the pattern of hyperpigmentation, PJS, AD, and Cushing's syndrome should also be considered. However, PJS does not have low blood pressure (hypotension) as part of its clinical presentation. Cushing syndrome is associated with hypertension therefore not a plausible option. AD has hypotension as part of its clinical manifestations. Therefore, the most likely cause for this patient's diffuse bilateral oral hyperpigmentation and persistent low blood pressure is AD. Measurement of ACTH activity via short corticotrophin test and plasma renin levels would help arrive at a definitive diagnosis of Addison disease.

Further reading

Alessandro L, Inam H, Letizia P, Antonio DE, Nicola C. Oral pigmentation as a sign of Addison's disease: a brief reappraisal. *The Open Dermatology Journal*, 2009;3(1):3–6.

83. A

The Hb$_{A1c}$ (glycosylated haemoglobin) is normal adult haemoglobin that binds to glucose and remains in the circulation for the life of the RBC. The Hb$_{A1c}$ is an important indicator of long-term glycaemic control with the ability to reflect the cumulative glycaemic history of the preceding 2–3 months. This ability permits its utilization as a longitudinal parameter, allowing patients to be monitored over years or even decades. The Hb$_{A1c}$ also correlates well with the risk of developing long-term diabetes complications. Elevated Hb$_{A1c}$ has also been regarded as an independent risk factor for coronary heart disease and stroke in subjects with or without diabetes. Diabetics are recommended to have a Hb1Ac test every 3–6 months. The Hb$_{A1c}$ result is given in a unit of measurement that is written as 'mmol/mol'. Previously it used to be given as a percentage (%). Its targets vary depending on the patient group (i.e. diabetics, non-diabetics, and patients at risk from the effects of hypoglycaemia). Therefore, a cumulative blood glucose in the preceding 3 months is the option which best depicts Hb1Ac.

Further reading

Wilkinson IB, Raine T, Wiles K, Goodhart A, Hall C, O'Neill H. Chapter 5: Endocrinology. In: Wilkinson IB, *et al.* (eds). *Oxford Handbook of Clinical Medicine*, 10th Edition. Oxford, UK: Oxford University Press, 2019.

Infectious diseases

84. B

Glucose-6-phosphate dehydrogenase deficiency (G6PD) is a X-linked inherited disorder which is most prevalent in tropics and subtropics. Patients with G6PD develop are usually asymptomatic but can develop acute haemolytic anaemia when exposed to oxidative stress triggered by stressful periods, fava bean consumption, medications, or strenuous physical exercise. Examples of some medication that can trigger a crisis include chloroquine, primaquine, paracetamol, aspirin, and many more. Clinical features are those of acute haemolytic anaemia (i.e. pallor, jaundice, fatigue, splenomegaly, and dark urine) and favism if related to fava beans consumption and chronic non-spherocytic haemolytic anaemia.

Pyruvate kinase (PK) deficiency, transmitted as an autosomal recessive trait, is the most frequent enzyme abnormality of the glycolytic pathway, and the most common cause of hereditary non-spherocytic haemolytic anaemia. Clinical manifestations of PK deficiency comprise the usual hallmarks of lifelong chronic haemolysis. The routine haematological laboratory features of PK deficiency are common to other hereditary non-spherocytic haemolytic diseases: anaemia of variable severity, reticulocytosis, and biochemical signs of hyperhaemolysis (i.e. increased unconjugated bilirubin concentrations).

Sickle cell disease is inherited as an autosomal-dominant trait, individuals who are heterozygous for the β^S allele carry the sickle cell trait (HbAS) but do not have sickle cell disease, whereas individuals who are homozygous for the β^S allele have sickle cell anaemia (HbSS). The sickle Hb (HbS) allele, β^S, is an *HBB* allele in which an adenine-to-thymine substitution results in the replacement of glutamic acid with valine at position 6 in the mature β-globin chain. Under conditions of deoxygenation (that is, when the Hb is not bound to oxygen), Hb tetramers that include two of these mutant sickle β-globin subunits (that is, HbS) can polymerize and cause the erythrocytes to assume a crescent or sickled shape. Sickle erythrocytes can lead to chronic haemolytic anaemia, recurrent vaso-occlusive episodes resulting in unpredictable episodes of pain and widespread organ damage, all of which are hallmarks of sickle cell disease.

Spherocytosis is a hereditary condition which manifests as haemolytic anaemia. It is caused by a defect in RBC membrane which results in destabilization of the membrane leading to RBC, assuming an abnormal morphology (spherical shape), having a reduced lifespan (from 120 days to a few days), i.e. increased haemolysis. The clinical features range from asymptomatic to the severe presentation. It manifests as the classical clinical features of haemolysis (i.e. anaemia, splenomegaly, jaundice). Laboratory investigation will reveal reticulocytosis, spherocytes on blood film, and raised unconjugated bilirubin (jaundice).

The clinical features (headache, malaise, and jaundice) and blood tests findings (normocytic anaemia, raised reticulocyte count, and raised unconjugated bilirubin) are classical clinical features of haemolysis, irrespective of the cause. Therefore, all of the options are plausible as they all can cause defects in RBCs which make them susceptible to early breakdown. However, considering this patient only developed their clinical features on return from a trip to Zanzibar in Tanzania, the hereditary causes of haemolytic anaemia (G6PD and PK deficiency, sickle cell disease, and hereditary spherocytosis) are highly unlikely to be plausible options. That leaves us with malaria, a protozoan infection endemic in Zanzibar, Tanzania. In malaria, the plasmodium species introduced by the Anopheles mosquito invades RBCs and initiates a cycle of cell lysis and further parasitization. This invasion and the metabolic activity of the parasite alter the RBC membrane resulting in splenic sequestration and massive RBC haemolysis, hence the manifestation as a haemolytic anaemia. The patient is likely to have become infected from mosquito bites during their visit.

Further reading

Dhaliwai G, Cornett PA, Tierney LM. Hemolytic anaemia. *Am Fam Physician*, 2004;69:2599–608.

85. E

Cervical lymphadenopathy, painless firm tongue ulcer and a history of a healed genital ulcer suggest this patient may still have primary syphilis or is on the verge of transiting into secondary syphilis. The healed genital ulcer may represent the chancre which develops at the site of infection.

Establishing a diagnosis is usually based on a constellation of clinical history, symptom presentation, and direct and serologic test results.

Dark field microscopy is the most specific technique for diagnosing syphilis when an active chancre or condylomata (found in moist areas between body folds) is present. It is a direct detection technique which involves collecting scrapings of the sore, placing it on a slide and examining under a dark field microscope. Dark field microscopy from specimens obtained in the mouth or anogenital region can generate false-positive results because normal non-pathogenic treponemes which are indistinguishable microscopically from *T. pallidum* exist at these sites. The genital ulcer is healed in this patient, hence scrapings required for dark field microscopy cannot be collected. Of note, dark field microscopy also requires levels of skill and experience that are no longer common pathology laboratories in developed countries.

Microbiology and culture are not a plausible option, because *Treponema pallidum* is too fragile an organism to be cultured in the clinical setting.

Because of how thin *Treponema pallidum* is, it is difficult to classify its Gram stain. Therefore, Gram staining is also not a plausible option.

Utilization of polymerase chain reaction test for detection of *Treponema pallidum* DNA have been demonstrated in many research studies. However, it is not currently an established clinical diagnostic test.

There are two types of diagnostic blood tests: treponemal and non-treponemal tests.

A non-treponemal test includes venereal disease research laboratory (VDRL) or rapid plasma reagin (RPR) test. Both measure the host's response to non-treponemal antigen such as cardiolipin and lecithin released from the damaged host cells. They also measure lipoprotein-like material released from the treponema. Both tests are considered sensitive in early syphilis but can suffer false-positive in patient with autoimmune disease, collagen disease, and leprosy. False negative in early and late latent syphilis due to reduced sensitivity is reported. The result is given in titres.

Treponemal tests include fluorescent treponemal antibody absorbed (FTA-ABS), *Treponema pallidum* particle agglutination (TP-PA), enzyme immunoassay (EIA), chemiluminescence immunoassay (CIA). These tests have high sensitivity for all the stages of disease other than very early primary syphilis. They detect human serum/plasma antibodies to *Treponema pallidum* by means of an indirect hemagglutination method. The results of these tests are given as either 'positive' or 'negative'.

Considering there is no information on the pregnancy status of the patient, the presence of autoimmune disorders or infections, all of which can generate a false-positive result with the non- treponemal tests. The most likely investigation to be of diagnostic value in this patient is the RPR test. In practice, a positive non-treponemal test result is usually followed-up by testing with a treponemal test to confirm the positive result. It is worth remembering that the treponemal-based tests remain positive for life and cannot distinguish between recent, active infection, and previously treated or old, non-contagious infection. Therefore, the result of these tests should not be interpreted without recourse to the patient clinical history, symptom presentation, and outcomes of other diagnostic tests.

Further reading

Grillo-Ardila CF, Angel-Müller E, Torres-Montañez NA, Vasquez-Velez LF, Amaya-Guio J. Point of care rapid test for diagnosis of syphilis infection in pregnant women. *Cochrane Database Syst Rev*, 2018;201 8(5):CD013037.

86. C

Infectious mononucleosis is caused by the EBV. The clinical findings of fever, malaise, sore throat, cervical lymphadenopathy, and palatal petechiae are consistent with infectious mononucleosis. However, because of the significant overlap of symptoms with other common viral illnesses and bacterial tonsillitis, testing as was carried out in this patient may be required to confirm a diagnosis of infectious mononucleosis. A positive monospot test indicates the presence of heterophile antibodies. This is in addition with the patient's symptoms is helpful in arriving at a diagnosis of infectious mononucleosis.

Despite high rates of specificity of the monospot test, false positives from other viral infections including cytomegalovirus, human immunodeficiency virus, rubella, and herpes simplex virus have been reported.

EBV is the most plausible option for the reasons elaborated here.

Further reading

Lennon P, Crotty M, Fenton JE. Infectious mononucleosis. *BMJ*, 2015;350:h1825.

87. E

Granulomatous inflammation is a distinctive form of chronic inflammation produced in response to various infectious, autoimmune, toxic, allergic, and neoplastic conditions. Common reaction patterns include necrotizing granulomas, non-necrotizing granulomas, suppurative granulomas, diffuse granulomatous inflammation, and foreign body giant cell reaction. The authors refer the readers to the further reading article for a detailed list of types of granulomas and associated aetiology.

Actinomycosis associated with exudation of pus containing sulphur granules produces suppurative granulomas hence not a plausible option.

Orofacial granulomatosis and sarcoidosis are both autoimmune conditions which cause non-necrotizing granulomas. Therefore, both are not plausible options.

Tuberculosis and granulomatosis with polyangiitis (Wegner's granulomatosis) are both associated with necrotizing granulomas.

Granulomatosis with polyangiitis is a vasculitic disorder which can affect upper respiratory tract, lower respiratory tract, and kidney. The severity of the disease can vary from an indolent disease affecting one site to a multiorgan vasculitis. Patients usually have antibodies to cytoplasmic component of neutrophils (ANCA). The key histologic features include necrotizing vasculitis involving small vessels, extensive geographic necrosis, and granulomatous inflammation.

Tuberculosis (TB) is an infectious condition caused by mycobacterium tuberculosis. The classical clinical features of active disease include chronic cough, haemoptysis, fever, night sweat, and weight loss. In the oral cavity, TB can present as a single, indurated, irregular, painless non-healing ulcer with associated regional lymphadenopathy. The tongue is the most commonly affected site, however involvement of other sites including the palate, lips, buccal mucosa, gingiva have been described. Note, the oral presentation is usually non-specific, thus a diagnosis is only reached if a biopsy of lesion shows classic necrotizing granuloma or when a diagnosis of pulmonary tuberculosis is established.

The constellations of the patient's clinical findings (i.e. a non-healing tongue ulcer, cervical lymphadenopathy, night sweats, weight loss and nocturnal fever) make tuberculosis the most likely cause of the patient's oral finding.

Further reading

Shah KK, Pritt BS, Alexander MP. Histopathologic review of granulomatous inflammation. *Journal of Clinical Tuberculosis and Other Mycobacterial Diseases,* 2017;7:1–2.

Psychiatry in dentistry

88. C

Options A, B, D, and E are clinical features suggestive of a diagnosis of depression. Bipolar affective disorder (BAD) or manic depression typically involves prolonged episodes of depression which alternate with periods of mania (i.e. significantly elevated mood). Affected patients may also demonstrate irritability. Characteristic clinical features of mania include increased energy, pressure of speech, increased self-esteem, reduced need for sleep, increased sex drive, and reckless behaviour including excessive spending or gambling without considering the consequences. This behaviour can seriously affect the patient's health, work, personal, and family life. Between episodes of depression and mania, affected patients will have stable mood. Both morbidity and mortality in BAD are high and affected patients may attempt suicide often during an episode of depression.

Further reading

Semple D, Smyth R. Chapter 8: Bipolar illness. In: Semple D, Smyth R (eds). *Oxford Handbook of Psychiatry*, 3rd Edition. Oxford, UK: Oxford University Press, 2013.

89. D

Obsessive-compulsive disorder (OCD) is a common chronic distressing disorder which frequently first occurs before the age of 25 years. It often generates considerable anxiety and may lead to depression. Obsessions may be defined as 'recurring, persisting, and distressing thoughts, images or impulses which the affected patient recognizes as their own but may recognize them to be unreasonable or excessive'. This patient has repeated intrusive obsessive thoughts regarding bad breath (oral malodour). Obsessional thoughts typically generate distressing anxiety which may be relieved by related compulsions (which may be thought of as the 'motor' component of obsessional thoughts). In this case the patient is toothbrushing and using mouthwashes frequently. OCD themes are numerous but may include 'checking', 'washing', and concerns about contamination. *Note*: this patient is not attributing the oral malodour to possible disease which would be characteristic of hypochondriasis, rather they are taking compulsive actions to alleviate persisting thoughts. However, like hypochondriasis, the patient has made persistent attempt to seek information and reassurance about the oral malodour from healthcare practitioners.

Further reading

Semple D, Smyth R. Chapter 9: Anxiety and stress-related disorders. In: Semple D, Smyth R (eds). *Oxford Handbook of Psychiatry*, 3rd Edition. Oxford, UK: Oxford University Press, 2013.

90. D

Ongoing, significantly reduced interest or enjoyment in most or all activities so-called 'anhedonia' is a fundamental symptom of depression. Depressed patients typically experience fatigue, altered sleeping patterns with difficulty getting off to sleep and early morning wakening such that they wake unrefreshed, weight change, reduced sexual drive, diminished concentration, and feelings of hopeless, helplessness, and lack of worth. Options A and E are suggestive of schizophrenia. Option B suggests hypothyroidism. Symptoms and clinical features suggestive of hypothyroidism include fatigue, weakness, lowered mood, weight gain, constipation, reduced memory, and dementia. Option C suggests dementia. Therefore option D is the most plausible option.

Further reading

Semple D, Smyth R. Chapter 7: Depressive illness. In: Semple D, Smyth R (eds). *Oxford Handbook of Psychiatry*, 3rd Edition. Oxford, UK: Oxford University Press, 2013.

91. D

An anaphylactic attack is a severe, life-threatening, generalized, or systemic hypersensitivity reaction. Clinical features include, urticaria, erythema, rhinitis, conjunctivitis, abdominal pain, vomiting, diarrhoea, flushing, pallor, stridor, wheezing, hoarse voice, collapse etc. Patient would require treatment with intramuscular injection of adrenaline, 0.5 ml of 1:1,000 for symptoms to resolve.

Asthmatic attack is a localized hypersensitivity reaction that affects the airway. Clinical features depend on whether it an acute severe or life-threatening asthma, they include wheezing, inability to complete sentences, tachycardia, increased respiratory rate, cyanosis, etc. Resolution of symptoms would require treatment with salbutamol inhaler which is a short-acting β_2 adrenal receptor agonist.

Epileptic attack is characterized by the grand-mal (tonic-clonic) seizures (i.e. an aura, sudden loss of consciousness, rigidity, and cyanosis, jerking movement of the limbs, frothing, and urinary incontinence). Seizures are self-limiting in that they typically last a few minutes then patient recover consciousness and become floppy.

Syncopal attack refers to a transient loss of consciousness which is most commonly caused by vagal overactivity. Clinical features include patient feels faint/light-headed, bradycardia, pallor, sweating, nausea, and vomiting, etc. Management is by laying the patient flat as soon as possible and raise legs to improve venous returns.

Panic attack which is the most likely cause of this patient symptoms implies a discrete period of intense fear or discomfort that is of sudden onset, and rapidly builds up to peak usually over 10 minutes or less. This is often accompanied by a sense of imminent danger or impending doom. It is characterized by a wide range of symptoms and signs caused by autonomic nervous system stimulation. It is not uncommon for patient with dental and/or needle phobias to experience panic attacks in a dental setting. In the longer term this patient may benefit from recommended psychological interventions such as breathing retraining, cognitive restructuring, interceptive exposure, and relaxation training. In the short term, the affected phobic patient may benefit from sedation.

Panic attack is the most plausible option.

Further reading

Semple D, Smyth R. Chapter 9: Anxiety and stress-related disorders. In: Semple D, Smyth R (eds). *Oxford Handbook of Psychiatry*, 3rd Edition. Oxford, UK: Oxford University Press, 2013.

92. C

Risk factors for suicide include:

- Family history of suicide
- Family history of child maltreatment
- Previous suicide attempts
- History of mental disorder particularly clinical depression
- History of alcohol and substance
- Feeling of hopelessness
- Impulsive or aggressive tendencies
- Isolation
- Loss (divorce, social, work, or financial)
- Easy access to lethal methods
- Barrier to accessing mental health
- Cultural and religious belief (belief that suicide is a noble resolution of a personal dilemma)

Protective factors which buffer individuals from suicidal thoughts and behaviour include:

- Skills in problem solving, conflict resolution, non-violent ways of handling disputes
- Cultural and religious belief that discourage suicide and support instincts for self-preservation
- Support for medical and mental health
- Family and community support (connectedness)
- Easy access to a variety of clinical interventions and support for help seeking
- Effective clinical care
- Hopefulness
- Good skills in problem-solving
- Responsibility for children

Cultural and religious beliefs may act as both a risk and protective factor in different individuals; this is because different cultures and religions have different views on suicide, as highlighted here. Therefore, connectedness to family and community support is the most plausible answer from the aforementioned options.

Further reading

Centers for Disease Control and Prevention. *Risk and Protective Factors: Risk Factors for Suicide.* Available at: https://www.cdc.gov/violenceprevention/suicide/riskprotectivefactors.html

Thomas J, Monaghan T. Chapter 16: The psychiatric assessment. In: Thomas J, Monaghan T (eds). *Oxford Handbook of Clinical Examination and Practical Skills*, 2nd Edition. Oxford, UK: Oxford University Press, 2014.

93. B

A 'hallucination' is defined as a perception which arises in the absence of any external stimulus. A 'delusion' is defined as a false belief which is steadfastly held in spite of evidence to the contrary. A delusion is typically bizarre and is unrelated to the affected patient's cultural or educational background. Delusions, including delusions of control and interference with thinking such as thought insertion, withdrawal or broadcasting and auditory hallucinations particularly of voices are described as 'positive' or 'acute' symptoms of schizophrenia and are included in the so-called first rank symptoms of schizophrenia. Visual hallucinations typically occur in organic psychiatric states. Delusions may occur in a wide variety of conditions including severe depression where they are typically 'mood congruent' (e.g. of poverty or guilt). They can occur in isolation as a so-called monosymptomatic delusional disorder (e.g. delusions of infestation such as Ekbom syndrome).

Hallucination is the most plausible option.

Further reading

Semple D, Smyth R. Chapter 3: Symptoms of psychiatric illness. In: Semple D, Smyth R (eds). *Oxford Handbook of Psychiatry*, 3rd Edition. Oxford, UK: Oxford University Press, 2013.

Immunological diseases

94. C

There are five classes of immunoglobulin, IgM, IgG, IgA, IgD, and IgE.

IgM antibodies are associated with primary immune response and are used to diagnose acute exposure to a pathogen.

IgG antibodies are the predominant isotype found in the body. There are four subtypes IgG1, IgG2, IgG3, and IgG4. IgG1 to IgG3 play a role in activating the complement cascade which results in the clearance of opsonized pathogens.

IgA is associated with mucosal surfaces and found in secretions (i.e. saliva and breast milk). There are two subclasses IgA1 and IgA2. IgA plays a critical role in protecting mucosal surfaces from toxins, virus, and bacteria.

IgD is found at very low levels in serum. Its function is unclear.

IgE is a very potent antibody which is present at low serum levels. It is associated with hypersensitivity and allergic reactions as well as the response to parasitic worm infections.

The dry skin with erythema and scaling, constant itching, hyperpigmented, or hypopigmented affected areas are characteristic of eczema. In chronic eczema, the skin can become thickened and lichenified. Peripheral IgE levels may be elevated in eczema, but this is not a standard test for the diagnosis. Based on the aforementioned points, IgE immunoglobulin is certainly the most likely to be out of range in this patient.

Further reading

Schroeder Jr HW, Cavacini L. Structure and function of immunoglobulins. *J Allergy Clin Immunol*, 2010;125(2):S41–52.

95. D

Angio-oedema refers to transient painless swelling of subcutaneous or submucosal tissues in any part of the body due to increased vascular permeability. The swelling is usually non-pitting when pressure is applied. It can cause symptoms secondary to a pressure effect on neighbouring structures but can also lead to life-threatening complications when occurring in the airway. Angioedema can be mediated by histamine, bradykinin, and pseudoallergenic mechanisms or be idiopathic.

Histamine-mediated angioedema is also known as allergic angioedema. It is a type I IgE-mediated immediate hypersensitivity immune response caused by mast cell degranulation. Such reaction occurs following previous sensitization to the allergens.

Clinical features—Multisystemic manifestations including bronchospasm, urticaria, cutaneous flushing, and cardiac symptoms ranging from hypotension to cardiac arrest.

Treatment—Early administration of epinephrine (0.5 ml increments of 1:1,000 intramuscularly) is essential. Secondary treatments include steroids and antihistamines administration. Bronchodilators, salbutamol, can be used to relieve bronchospasm.

Bradykinin-mediated angioedema comprises three distinct types:

1. Hereditary angioedema—Arises from mutations in the gene encoding for C1 esterase inhibitor (C1-INH), resulting in either low plasma concentrations of C1-INH (HAE type I) or normal concentrations of functionally impaired C1-INH (HAE type II).

2. Acquired angioedema—Very rare, develops after the fourth decade and often associated with an underlying lymphoproliferative disorder.
3. ACE inhibitor (ACEi)-induced angioedema—Angiotensin-converting enzyme (ACE) breaks down bradykinin. ACE inhibitors will cause accumulation of bradykinin due to an impairment of carboxypeptidase N activity which is responsible for degrading bradykinin.

Treatment—Assess airway, if compromised, intubation, and emergency tracheostomy may be necessary. Treatment of the underlying cause by infusion of plasma derived or recombinant C1-estrase concentrate. Treatment with bradykinin receptor blocker icatibant or ecallantide (kallikrein inhibitor) may suffice.

Note: Histamine-mediated angioedema will respond to treatment with antihistamines, corticosteroids, and epinephrine, whereas bradykinin-mediated (including hereditary, acquired, and ACEi-induced) angioedema will not.

With this information, the most plausible option associated with the patient's swelling is hereditary angioedema which is a bradykinin-mediated angioedema caused by low C1 esterase inhibitor levels.

Further reading

Bernstein JA, Cremonesi P, Hoffmann TK, Hollingsworth J. Angioedema in the emergency department: a practical guide to differential diagnosis and management. *Int J Emerg Med,* 2017;10(1):15.

Hand manifestations of systemic diseases

96. B

See following brief description of finger and/or nail changes and their corresponding associated systemic conditions.

Osler's node refers to red, raised tender nodules on the pulps of toes or fingers.

Janeway lesion refers to a painless macule.

Splinter haemorrhages refer to linear haemorrhages lying parallel to the long axis of finger or toenails.

Osler's node, Janeway lesion, and splinter haemorrhages are associated with infective endocarditis.

Koilonychia (also known as spoon nails) refers to abnormally thin nails (usually of the hand) which have lost their convexity, becoming flat or even concave in shape—suggestive of iron deficiency anaemia.

Swan neck deformity refers to a deformed position of the finger in which the middle joint of a finger is extended (bent back) more than normal and the end joint is flexed (bent down)—suggestive of rheumatoid arthritis.

Tendon xanthomata refers to freely mobile papules or nodules in the tendons, ligaments, fascia, and periosteum especially on the back of hands, fingers, elbows, knees, and heels— suggestive of familial hypercholesterolemia

Terry's nail (Leukonychia) refers to white nails, the nail beds become opaque, leaving only a rim of pink nail bed at the top of nail. It is usually caused hypoalbuminaemia of chronic liver disease, but can also be associated with fungal infection, renal failure, and lymphoma.

Paronychia refers to inflammation involving the folds of tissue around the fingernail or toenail. Patients typically lose the cuticle of the nail, thus making the area between the nail fold and nail plate prone to bacterial and fungal invasion. Chronic paronychia may occur in association with eczema or psoriasis.

Finger clubbing is caused by increase in the soft tissue under the proximal nail plate of the distal part of the fingers or toes. This pushes the nail up, increasing the angle between the long axis of the nail and dorsal nail fold. This can approach 180 degrees in severe cases—it is associated with a wide range of conditions including lung cancer, bronchiectasis, lung abscess, cystic fibrosis, sarcoidosis, asbestosis, etc.; cardiovascular causes like infective endocarditis, congenital heart disease, etc.; hepatobiliary causes like primary biliary cirrhosis, cirrhosis of the liver associated chronic hepatitis B and C infection, alcohol misuse, and fatty liver disease. Gastrointestinal causes include ulcerative colitis, Crohn's disease, coeliac disease, etc.

Beau's lines refer to transverse/horizontal ridges or grooves in the nail plate that form as a result of temporary interference of cell division in the proximal nail matrix. The condition is self-limiting and can be associated with trauma, systemic illnesses including peripheral vascular disease, chemotherapeutic agents, etc.

The most likely finger/nail change to be associated with liver cirrhosis caused by alcohol and substance misuse is finger clubbing.

Further reading

Tan S, Senna MM. Hair and nail manifestations of systemic disease. *Curr Dermatol Rep,* 2017;6(1):17–28.

97. B

Plummer–Vinson (Paterson–Brown–Kelly) syndrome is rare and characterized by the triad of dysphagia, iron deficiency anaemia, and oesophageal webs. Historically, it was seen predominantly in in middle-aged women.

Indented spoon-shaped nails refer to koilonychia which is associated with iron deficiency anaemia.

Transverse grooves across the nails refers to Beau's line which can be associated with trauma, systemic illnesses including peripheral vascular disease, chemotherapeutic agents, etc.

White nails with reddened or dark tips refer to Terry's nails, which can be associated with liver cirrhosis, renal failure, lymphoma, etc.

Pitting/dents on the nails can be associated with psoriasis, eczema, reactive arthritis, and alopecia areata.

Brown streaks under the nails may represent splinter haemorrhages caused by lines of blood caused by tiny damaged blood vessels. Splinter haemorrhages can be associated with infective endocarditis.

The most plausible nail abnormalities seen in Plummer–Vinson syndrome is indented spoon-shaped nails (koilonychia) and it is caused by their iron deficiency anaemia.

Further reading

NI Direct. Nail abnormalities. Available at: https://www.nidirect.gov.uk/conditions/nail-abnormalities

Gastrointestinal diseases

98. A

The patient's clinical features including tummy aches, bloating, weight loss, tiredness, and mouth ulcers are suggestive of a lower gastrointestinal disorder. Because these symptoms are sufficiently similar for many lower gastrointestinal disorders, investigations to exclude conditions, and arrive at a definitive diagnosis are required.

Calprotectin is a protein released by neutrophils into stool when there is inflammation of the bowel. Raised faecal calprotectin indicates inflammation in the bowel but cannot establish the cause. For this reason, faecal calprotectin testing is used for distinguishing between IBD such as Crohn's disease, ulcerative colitis, coeliac disease, and non-IBDs such as IBS. To establish the cause of raised faecal calprotectin levels, further investigations are required. A raised antiendomysial antibody level (as seen in this patient) and a positive tissue transglutaminase (TTG) level are diagnostic of coeliac disease. This is particularly the case for children where a biopsy avoidance strategy is advocated. This strategy avoids the need for a gastroscopy, which often requires general anaesthesia in children. In other word, a raised TTG concentration higher than the upper limit of normal, positive EMA in a separate blood sample and the presence of HLA-DQ2 or HLA-DQ8 genotype is considered diagnostic in a symptomatic paediatric patient without the need for biopsy sampling. In adults, a combination of coeliac serology testing and duodenal biopsy sampling is required to establish a diagnosis. The characteristic duodenal biopsy features include intraepithelial lymphocytes, crypt hyperplasia, and villous atrophy.

Crohn's disease and ulcerative colitis are both IBD which cause raised faecal calprotectin. Finding raised antiendomysial antibody levels which is specific for coeliac disease, means both options are not plausible.

IBS is a functional disorder/non-IBD. Faecal calprotectin level and antiendomysial antibody level should be within normal range, therefore also not a plausible option.

Although symptomatic diverticular disease can also cause raised faecal calprotectin, antiendomysial antibody levels should be within normal range, hence not a plausible option.

Coeliac disease is the most plausible causes of this patient's features. It is triggered by ingestion of gluten in a genetically susceptible individual. It primarily affects the small intestine and presents diverse clinical manifestations including intestinal and extraintestinal features. They include chronic diarrhoea, failure to thrive, weight loss, bloating, constipation, iron deficiency anaemia, abdominal pain, osteoporosis, chronic fatigue, recurring headache, recurrent aphthous ulceration, etc.

Further reading

Lebwohl B, Sanders DS, Green PH. Coeliac disease. *Lancet*, 2018;391(10115):70–81.

National Institute for Health and Care Excellence. Faecal calprotectin diagnostic tests for inflammatory diseases of the bowel. Diagnostics guidance [DG11]. Available at: https://www.nice.org.uk/guidance/dg11

99. D

The Troisier's sign represents an enlarged left-sided supraclavicular lymph node. The enlarged supraclavicular lymph node is also known as a Virchow node (VN), Troisier node, or Virchow–Troisier node. In the mid-to-late nineteenth century, an enlarged supraclavicular node was thought to be a clinical sign of gastric cancer metastasis. The VN is now known as a seeding location for cancers arising from myriad locations apart from the stomach, including the intestines, urogenital system, oesophagus, common bile duct, liver, as well as the pancreas, and lungs. The VN has also been reported with squamous cell carcinoma and lymphoma. This association with a wide range of malignancies can be attributed to its location at the junction of the thoracic duct and the left subclavian vein, where the lymph from most of the body drains into the systemic circulation. The finding of Virchow's node indicates advanced disease.

Gastric adenocarcinoma is the most plausible option considering it well established associated with the enlarged left supraclavicular lymph node (Virchow's node).

Further reading

Siosaki MD, Souza AT. Virchow's node. *N Engl J Med*, 2013;368:e7.

100. C

Traditional markers which can be used to assess a person's alcohol intake (i.e. history of heavy drinking) or whether they have had a recent binge include gamma-glutamyl transpeptidase (GGT), aspartate transaminase (AST), alanine transaminase (ALT), MCV, and carbohydrate-deficient transferrin (CDT).

Raised GGT is seen in alcoholics but can also be an indicator of early liver disease, pancreatitis, obesity, and prostate disease. It has a sensitivity of 61%. ALT and AST are both raised in alcoholics but are less sensitive measures of alcoholism compared to GGT. Comparatively, ALT is a more specific measure of alcohol induced liver injury compared to AST which is also found in other organs including liver, brain, muscle, heart, and kidneys. The ratio AST/ALT is a better marker of chronic alcohol abuse or chronic liver damage compared ALT and AST in isolation. Raised MCV is associated with heavy drinking. The association of raised MCV with other conditions (pernicious anaemia, folate deficiency anaemia, hypothyroidism, etc.) reduces its specificity and can further confound its interpretation. CDT is elevated in heavy alcohol abuse. CDT is far more specific than GGT and other liver function tests. While all of these markers can be raised in an alcoholic patient, an elevated GGT remains the most widely used marker of alcohol abuse, therefore the most plausible option.

Further reading

Strid N, Litten RZ. *Assessing Alcohol Problems: A Guide for Clinicians and Researchers.* NIH Publications, 2003;3:37. Available at: https://pubs.niaaa.nih.gov/publications/assessingalcohol/

Renal diseases

101. C

Nephrotic syndrome is a characterized by glomerular defects which manifests as large amounts of protein into urine. Clinical manifestations include oedema which is typically pitting and dependent. The oedema can also occur around and in the periorbital area because tissue resistance here is low. Urine dipstick test usually reveals massive proteinuria while blood test can show low albumin levels and hyperlipidaemia.

Nephritic syndrome is caused by inflammation of the glomerulus which results in a thin glomerular basement membrane and small pores, large enough to permit proteins and RBCs to pass into urine. It is a manifestation of different conditions including infectious, autoimmune, or thrombotic. Typical examples include post streptococcal glomerulonephritis, IgA nephropathy, systemic lupus erythematous, etc. Clinical features include blood in urine (haematuria), protein in urine (proteinuria), hypertension, low urine output, blurred vision, increase in blood creatinine and blood urea nitrogen.

Polycystic kidney disease is slowly progressing hereditary kidney disease characterized by the progressive development of bilateral renal cysts, resulting in urine concentration defects, enlargement of the kidney volume due to cystic formations, hypertension, haematuria, acute and chronic pain, cyst and urinary tract infections, and loss of renal function. It is a multisystemic disease with several extrarenal manifestations including hepatic cysts, pancreatic cysts, intracranial aneurysms, colon diverticulosis, and heart valve defects.

Acute interstitial nephritis also known as acute tubulointerstitial nephritis is characterized by inflammation involving the interstitium and tubules of the kidney. Causes include drug-induced, infection-associated, and cases associated with immune or neoplastic disorders. Clinical features include malaise, anorexia, nausea, and vomiting, increased creatinine and blood urea nitrogen.

Urinary tract infection refers to infection that affects part of the urinary tract. In the bladder it is referred to as cystitis, and in the kidney as pyelonephritis. Clinical features of cystitis include pain on micturition, frequent urination, etc. Pyelonephritis can present with fever, malaise, and flank pain.

Considering there is no mention of haematuria (nephritic syndrome, polycystic kidney disease), cystic changes in the kidney or elsewhere (polycystic kidney disease), changes to blood urea nitrogen and creatinine, decrease urine output (tubulointerstitial nephritis and nephritic syndrome), pain on micturition, frequent urination, malaise, flank pain (urinary tract infection) in this patient, the most plausible option is nephrotic syndrome.

Further reading

Wilkinson IB, Raine T, Wiles K, Goodhart A, Hall C, O'Neill H. Chapter 7: Renal medicine. In: Wilkinson IB, *et al.* (eds). *Oxford Handbook of Clinical Medicine*, 10th Edition. Oxford, UK: Oxford University Press, 2019.

102. B

End-stage renal failure can result in a range of clinical manifestations affecting virtually all body systems. Some of the clinical manifestations and their corresponding pathophysiological mechanisms can be seen in Table 2.8.

Table 2.8 Clinical manifestations of end-stage renal disease and their corresponding pathophysiological mechanisms

Clinical manifestations	Possible pathophysiological mechanisms
Normocytic normochromic anaemia (low haemoglobin)	1. Failure of renal production of erythropoietin 2. Toxic suppression of bone marrow 3. Increased red cell fragility 4. Renal loss of RBC
Purpura and bleeding tendency	1. Impaired platelet adhesiveness 2. Diminished platelet thromboxane production 3. Defective and decreased Von Willebrand factor 4. Raised prostacyclin levels
Bone pain (renal osteodystrophy)	1. Raised phosphate level 2. Decreased calcium level 3. Raised parathyroid hormone 4. Deficiency of renal production of 1,25 dlhydroxycholecalciferol (vitamin D)
Hypertension	1. Impaired sodium and water excretion 2. Activation of the renin-angiotensin system 3. Sympathetic activation
Increased chance of malignancies ranging from lymphomas to skin cancers (i.e. basal cell and squamous cell carcinomas)	1. Immunosuppression
Giant cell/Browns tumour	1. Secondary hyperparathyroidism

Brown tumour attributable to secondary hyperparathyroidism is the most plausible option.

Further reading

Gadhia T, Adegun OK, Fortune F. Brown tumours: widespread involvement of multiple maxillofacial bones and cervical spine. *Case Rep*, 2014;2014:bcr2014207140.

Greenwood M, Meechan JG, Bryant DG. General medicine and surgery for dental practitioners part 7: renal disorders. *Br Dent J*, 2003;195:181–4.

Respiratory diseases

103. B

A spacer device is a large plastic empty device with openings at both ends, one end unto which a pressured metered dose inhaler (pMDI) is inserted and the opposite end, a mouthpiece which inserts into the patient's mouth. Some mouth pieces incorporate a unidirectional valve which allows for inhalation but not exhalation into the spacer. The use of spacer devices negates the critical problem of poor coordination of activation of the pMDI with commencement of inhalation typically seen in children, the elderly, patients with compromised manual dexterity and in a medical emergency situation.

Advantages of using a spacer device:

- Slow down the aerosol as it emerges from the pMDI
- Reduces the impact of hand-breath coordination problems
- Reduces oropharyngeal impaction/deposition and local side effects (oral candidiasis, when inhaled corticosteroids are used)
- Reduces fraction of swallowed drug, gastrointestinal absorption, systemic bioavailability and thus extrapulmonary unwanted effects (β-adrenergic agonists)
- Improved lung deposition
- Allows for more inhalation time

Disadvantages:

- Require regular cleaning
- Can be rather bulky and less portable
- Electrostatic charge may reduce the respirable aerosol fraction

Considering this patient is not experiencing an acute asthmatic episode, the need for hand–breath coordination which is beneficial in the very young and elderly patients and in patients with poor manual dexterity does not represent best benefit a spacer device would confer.

There is no mention of the age of the patient, therefore reduced requirement for good manual dexterity as the sole benefit for its use is not a plausible option.

Reduced respirable aerosol fraction of steroids due to electrostatic charge is not a benefit of using spacer devices, therefore not a plausible option.

Reduced systemic bioavailability can be a benefit of using spacer device in this patient as it will help to minimize gastrointestinal absorption and unwanted extrapulmonary side effect of steroids. The bulky and less portable nature of a spacer device is however not a benefit. The latter makes this option not plausible.

A spacer device has an advantage of reducing the deposition/impaction of steroids on the soft palate and oropharynx, thereby minimizing the chances of developing local side effects (i.e. oral candidiasis). Considering this patient already suffers recurrent oral thrush, the recommendation of a spacer device use will further reduce oropharyngeal deposition of inhaled corticosteroid and stop/reduce this side effect. Therefore, this option best represents the benefits of using a spacer device in this patient.

Further reading

Vincken W, Levy ML, Scullion J, Usmani OS, Dekhuijzen PR, Corrigan CJ. Spacer devices for inhaled therapy: why use them, and how? *ERJ Open Res*, 2018;4(2):00065–2018.

104. C

Bronchiectasis is a progressive respiratory disease characterized by permanent dilatation of the bronchi and associated with a clinical syndrome of cough, sputum production, and recurrent respiratory infections. Recognized aetiologies include post-infection, chronic obstructive pulmonary disease (COPD), primary ciliary dyskinesia (PCD), allergic bronchopulmonary aspergillosis (ABPA), non-tuberculous mycobacterial infections, immune deficiencies, and connective tissue diseases. Bronchiectasis patient usually have a history of chronic cough which progressively worsen over the years. Exacerbation by recurrent respiratory infection with *Pseudomonas aeruginosa* is characteristic. Patient can also present weight loss and fatigue and fever but are unlikely to present axillary lymphadenopathy.

Clinical features of COPD include cough, expectoration of sputum, shortness of breath upon exertion or lower respiratory tract infections occurring more frequently or lasting longer than expected (>2 weeks). Identification of risk factors such as exposure to cigarette smoke, environmental or occupational pollutants, and/or the presence of a family history of obstructive lung diseases in association with these clinical features also raise the suspicion of COPD. Advanced disease can result in increased respiratory rate with forced expiratory efforts, decreased breath sounds on chest auscultation, the presence of rhonchi (rattling sounds), coarse crackles and wheezes and, in the most advanced cases, cyanosis (blue skin discolouration, a sign of hypoxaemia) might be present and should be considered an important complication that requires therapy with oxygen. A diagnosis of COPD is confirmed by a spirometer which demonstrates expiratory airflow limitation during a forced expiratory manoeuvre from total lung capacity to residual volume.

Pulmonary embolism most commonly originates from deep venous thrombosis of the legs, ranges from asymptomatic, incidentally discovered emboli to massive embolism causing immediate death. Pulmonary embolism should be suspected in all patients who present with new or worsening dyspnoea, chest pain, or sustained hypotension without an alternative obvious cause. Other clinical features include sudden onset or evolving over a period of days to weeks of cough, palpitations, and light-headedness, fever, and wheezing. The clinical feature correlates with the degree of the thromboembolic burden (i.e. large thrombi in the periphery may evolve silently and then present as symptomatic or even fatal pulmonary embolism, whereas smaller emboli may be associated with major symptoms, particularly if cardiovascular reserve is already poor). Risk factors for pulmonary embolism are advancing age, pregnancy, sedentary lifestyle, major surgery, trauma, cancer, oral contraceptive pills, hormone replacement therapy, obesity.

Pulmonary oedema refers accumulation of extravascular fluid in the lungs, which may develop from cardiogenic or non-cardiogenic causes. Cardiogenic causes include a variety of left side heart disorders including coronary artery disease, myocardiopathies, aortic or mitral valve abnormalities, all of which causes an increase pulmonary capillary hydrostatic pressure. Non-cardiogenic causes arise from injury to the lung sufficient to increase endothelial permeability and causes extravasation of proteinaceous fluid into the interstitium and alveolar spaces. Causes include lung injury, direct (inhalation of corrosive gases, gastric aspiration) or indirect (sepsis, pancreatitis, pneumonia, multiple trauma). Clinical features of both overlap; they include shortness of breath, tachypnoea, and hypoxia.

Lung cancer can broadly into to non-small cell lung cancer (NSCLC) and small cell lung cancer. Three main types of NSCLC are adenocarcinoma, squamous cell carcinoma, and large cell carcinoma. Early lung cancer is largely asymptomatic, and internalization of tumours means patients may not be alerted by obvious physical changes. When established, lung cancer can present with cough, haemoptysis (20% of cases), chest and shoulder pain, dyspnoea, hoarseness, weight loss, anorexia, fever, weakness, and bone pain. The clinical features are caused by the local tumour, intrathoracic spread, distant metastases, or paraneoplastic syndromes.

While the presence of cough, sputum production, and dyspnoea is not specific to any respiratory disease, the possibility of lung cancer should be suspected in a symptomatic patient the age of 50 years with a history of smoking. In this patient, the presence of progressive loss of appetite, weight loss, haemoptysis, finger clubbing, and axillary lymphadenopathy, the short duration since the onset of clinical features (<8 weeks) and the duration of exposure to a known risk factor (i.e. 35 years pack history of cigarette smoking) overwhelmingly favours the diagnosis of lung cancer over the other proffered diagnoses.

Further reading

BMJ Best Practice. Available at: http://bestpractice.bmj.com/best-practice/monograph/1082/diagnosis/step-by-step.html

105. C

Asking questions during the medical history can help determine the background chronic asthma severity and the severity of the acute attack.

Predictors or markers of chronic asthma severity and severity of acute episodes include:

- Recent hospital admission
- Three or more regular medications
- Frequent after hour general practitioner visits
- Previous ever intensive care unit admissions
- Heavy use of β_2 agonist
- Precipitate asthma
- Marked (>50%) reduction or variation in peak flow

Concurrent use of two medications for asthma is not a plausible option as most asthmatics use both brown 'steroid' and blue 'salbutamol' inhalers for prophylaxis and management of acute asthmatic episodes respectively. Exacerbation of asthma by exercise is not a plausible option because patient can experience this feature irrespective of their asthma severity. Previous life-threatening asthma attack (ever), necessitating previous intensive care unit (ICU) admission best identifies a patient at long-term risk of death. Marked variability in peak flow (i.e. morning dips) can be a good predictor of the severity of asthma attack only if monitored regularly. Sensitivity to paracetamol is rare hence not a plausible option. A hospital admission for an asthmatic episode during the last year is the most plausible option because it is reliable and easily ascertained.

Further reading

Aldington S, Beasley R. Asthma exacerbations. 5: Assessment and management of severe asthma in adults in hospital. *Thorax*, 2007;62(5):447–58.

106. B

Various clinical symptoms and signs can assist in determining the severity of acute asthma. Please refer to figure 1 in the further reading reference for a detailed characterization of the clinical signs and symptoms indicative of the different acute asthma severity. This table provides guidance as to what clinical symptoms and signs are associated with mild, moderate, and severe asthma. It also provides clinical findings which may suggest a respiratory arrest may be imminent.

Tachycardia and tachypnoea are both associated with severe acute asthma, therefore both are not plausible options.

Talking in sentences, phrases, and words are associated with mild, moderate, and severe acute asthma, respectively. Therefore, talking in words is not a plausible option.

Moderate wheeze, often only in end expiration is associated with mild acute asthma, loud wheeze throughout exhalation with moderate acute asthma and loud wheeze throughout inhalation and exhalation with severe acute asthma. An absence of wheeze suggests a respiratory arrest is imminent.

The use of accessory muscles is not unusual in moderate and severe acute asthma. However, the presence of paradoxical thoracoabdominal movements is highly indicative of an imminent respiratory arrest, and therefore is the most suitable option.

Further reading

Fergeson JE, Patel SS, Lockey RF. Acute asthma, prognosis, and treatment. *J Allergy Clin Immunol*, 2017;139(2):438–47.

107. A

COPD is characterized by persistent airflow limitation which is usually progressive and associated with an enhanced chronic inflammatory response in the airways and the lung to noxious particles or gases. The airflow limitation in COPD is largely irreversible owing to structural changes in the lungs (i.e. chronic obstructive bronchiolitis) due to fibrosis of small airways (<2-mm internal diameter), and emphysema, characterized by enlargement of alveoli and destruction of alveolar walls. Progressive airway obstructions lead to dyspnoea (shortness of breath on exertion) and, as a result, exercise limitation. COPD predominantly affects the elderly, with the peak prevalence at approximately 65 years of age and cigarette smoking, is the main risk factor. The main pathological features of COPD are obstructive bronchiolitis, emphysema and, in many cases, mucus hypersecretion (chronic bronchitis), therefore a diagnosis of COPD should be suspected in individuals with respiratory symptoms, such as cough, expectoration of sputum, shortness of breath upon exertion, or lower respiratory tract infections occurring more frequently or lasting longer than expected (>2 weeks). The suspicion should increase if the individuals also report risk factors for COPD, such as exposure to cigarette smoke, environmental or occupational pollutants, and/or the presence of a family history of obstructive lung diseases.

Patient with COPD can also experience night-time wheeze; however, their characteristic presentation is shortness of breath worsened by exertion which is due to progressive airway obstruction (obstructive bronchiolitis). Therefore, night-time wheeze in isolation is not a plausible option.

COPD risk strongly correlates with the inhalation of particulate matter from cigarette smoke and the burning of biomass for cooking or heating. Therefore, no history of smoking is not a plausible option.

COPD predominantly affects the elderly, with the peak prevalence at approximately 65 years of age. Therefore, the likelihood of symptoms first occurring in childhood as can occur in asthma is not the most likely option.

Variable severity of breathlessness (i.e. circadian variations of symptoms and lung function) is a well-known feature of asthma. While patients with COPD may experience some variation in the severity of their breathlessness, it is characteristically described as persistent and progressive. Therefore, this is also not the most plausible option.

Although the presence of cough, sputum production, or dyspnoea is not specific for COPD, in this scenario, chronic, productive cough is the most plausible option. It is due to mucus hypersecretion secondary to chronic bronchitis.

Further reading

Barnes PJ, Shapiro SD, Pauwels RA. Chronic obstructive pulmonary disease: molecular and cellular mechanisms. *Eur Resp J*, 2003;22(4):672–88.

Preoperative anaesthetic care

108. A

The Royal College of Surgeons of England defines a surgical day case as a patient who is admitted for investigations or operations on a planned non-resident basis and who nonetheless require facilities for recovery. Day-case surgery and outpatient cases are not synonymous. Outpatient cases are minor procedures carried out under local anaesthesia which do not generally require postoperative recovery time. The term '23-hour stay' in the UK is considered in patient care. Patient assessment for day-case surgery falls into three main categories: social, medical, and surgical.

- Social factors:
  - Patient must understand the planned procedure and postoperative care and give informed consent to day surgery.
  - It is essential that following procedures under general or regional anaesthesia, a responsible adult should escort the patient home. However, it may not be essential for a carer to remain for the full 24-hour period.
- Medical factors:
  - Fitness for a procedure should relate to the patient's functional status as determined at preanaesthetic assessment and not by American Society of Anesthesiologists (ASA) physical status, age, or body mass index. Patient with stable chronic disease can be treated with day-case surgery because there is minimal disruption to their daily routine. Those with unstable medical conditions are contraindicated from having day-case surgery.
  - Obesity is not a contraindication to day case surgery. Obese patient can be safely managed if appropriate resources are available.
  - Obstructive sleep apnoea is not an absolute contraindication to day surgery.
- Surgical factors:
  - The procedure must not carry a significant risk of serious postoperative complications requiring immediate medical attention (e.g. haemorrhage or cardiovascular instability).
  - Postoperative symptoms such as pain and nausea must be controllable by the use of a combination of oral medications and local anaesthetic techniques.
  - The procedure should not prohibit the patient from resuming oral intake within a few hours of the end of surgery.
  - Patient should be able to mobilize before discharge. If full mobilization is not possible, appropriate venous thromboembolism prophylaxis should be instituted and maintained.

With this background, angina at rest, an unstable chronic medical condition is the most likely option to make this patient unsuitable for wisdom tooth extraction under general anaesthesia as a day-case surgery. The other options are not contraindications to performing the wisdom tooth extraction under general anaesthesia.

Further reading

Bailey CR, et al. Guidelines for day-case surgery 2019: guidelines from the Association of Anaesthetists and the British Association of Day Surgery. *Anaesthesia*, 2019;74(6):778–92.

EXTENDED MATCHING QUESTIONS (EMQs)

Introduction

Students are less familiar with extended matching questions (EMQs) and find them particularly challenging to solve. This can be attributed to the layout of the question, the multiple options, and the statement which says, 'each option may be used once, more than once, or not at all'. Typically, EMQs are organized into a question theme, a list of 10 possible options followed by a set of items which can vary from clinical scenarios to drugs, etc. The correct answer to each item must be chosen from the list of options. It is hoped that the plethora of EMQs provided in this chapter would provide the readers particularly early year undergraduates several opportunities to familiarize themselves with this approach of testing knowledge.

Questions

1. Recognition of a patient's medication use

A. Beclomethasone inhaler

B. Betamethasone ointment

C. Chlorhexidine mouthwash

D. Difflam (benzydamine mouthwash)

E. Intravenous infusion of methylprednisolone

F. Intravenous infusion of zoledronate

G. Oral alendronate

H. Oral metformin 500 mg

I. Rivaroxaban

J. Subcutaneous injection of insulin

For each of the clinical scenarios described next, predict the SINGLE most likely medication you expect each patient to be using or have been prescribed from the previous list. Each option may be used once, more than once, or not at all.

1. A normal weight 20-year-old patient who developed diabetes at age 10 was administered intramuscular glucagon following an episode of unconsciousness at his last dental appointment.

2. A 45-year-old patient with multiple sclerosis presents with painful, erythematous, rhomboid-like area in the midline of the dorsum of the tongue. They have just had treatment for their disease which has exacerbated the oral soreness.

3. A 50-year-old patient with a history of bone metastases from breast cancer. She informs you of a previous consultation with the dentist, who recommended and commenced preventative measures before her current treatment was started.

4. A 55-year-old patient with atrial fibrillation had an emergency extraction of their wisdom tooth. The dentist applied Surgicel and sutured the tooth socket to control bleeding.

5. A 40-year-old patient with a history of gingival bleeding is concerned about the yellow discolouration of their teeth following the use of a recommended mouthwash which may be bought over the counter.

2. Recognition of a patient's morbidities

A. Addison's disease
B. Alcoholic liver disease
C. Erythema multiforme
D. Fatty liver disease
E. Hypothyroidism
F. Inflammatory bowel disease
G. Irritable bowel syndrome
H. Multiple sclerosis
I. Stevens–Johnson syndrome
J. Trigeminal neuralgia

For each of the patient scenarios described next, choose the SINGLE most likely morbidity each patient may be experiencing from the previous list. Each option may be used once, more than once, or not at all.

1. A 17-year-old patient presents with pyrexia, ocular redness. There is widespread oral ulceration, blood crusted lips, and target lesions on the skin. They are systemically unwell.

2. A 26-year-old patient complains of weight loss and has been experiencing recurrent abdominal pain associated with diarrhoea lasting more than 6 weeks. Their most recent blood and stool investigations revealed low haemoglobin and raised faecal calprotectin levels, respectively.

3. A 67-year-old patient with type II diabetes is grossly obese. They present with jaundice, generalized pruritus, bilateral ankle oedema, and upper right abdominal pain. Their social history is unremarkable. Blood investigations revealed abnormal liver function test.

4. A 34-year-old patient with a history of recent weight loss, lethargy, and low mood is concerned about recent episodes of unexplained diarrhoea and vomiting. Preliminary blood investigations reveal low blood glucose levels and hyperkalaemia.

5. A 40-year-old patient presents to the emergency department for sudden pain behind her left eye accompanied by blurred vision. Their recent past medical history is right-sided facial pain for which they have had multiple tooth extractions to relieve the symptoms.

3. **Therapeutics**

A. Amoxicillin
B. Cefalexin
C. Diclofenac
D. Ibuprofen
E. Metronidazole
F. Miconazole gel
G. Nifedipine
H. Nystatin suspension
I. Paracetamol
J. Ramipril

For each of the clinical scenarios described next, choose the SINGLE most likely medication necessary to manage each patient from the list, taking into account likely side effects, contraindications, and interactions. Each option may be used once, more than once, or not at all.

1. A patient with severe asthma and chronic rhinosinusitis requires postoperative pain relief after a tooth extraction.

2. A febrile alcoholic patient develops severe toothache complicated by a dentoalveolar abscess spreading into the floor of his mouth.

3. A patient on warfarin with a history of smoking requires treatment for oral candidiasis.

4. An atopic patient with a history of penicillin allergy requires antibiotic therapy for a spreading dentoalveolar abscess.

5. A hypertensive patient has recurrent episodes of oral ulceration since commencing treatment. Which medication may be associated with this?

4. **Cranial nerve abnormalities**

   A. Cranial nerve I
   B. Cranial nerve II
   C. Cranial nerve III
   D. Cranial nerve IV
   E. Cranial nerve V
   F. Cranial nerve VII
   G. Cranial nerve VIII
   H. Cranial nerve IX
   I. Cranial nerve XI
   J. Cranial nerve XII

   For each of the clinical scenarios described next, choose the SINGLE most likely cranial nerve involved from this list. Each option may be used once, more than once, or not at all.

   1. A patient presents at the emergency dental unit unable to close his mouth because this triggers a sharp electric-shock like and lancinating pain in the right upper lip. Administration of a right infraorbital nerve block provided immediate pain relief.

   2. A pensioner presents with sudden onset of blurred vision, severe pain in the left eye and surrounding area. On examination crops of tiny vesicles are beginning to appear in an area confined to the left forehead.

   3. A patient is concerned about sudden onset of hyperacusis. She has also noticed crops of tiny vesicles confined to the opening of their right ear.

   4. A patient presents with deviation of their jaw to opening.

   5. Following administration of an inferior dental nerve block to extract a mandibular right first molar, a patient becomes visibly distressed by drooling of saliva, inability to close the eye and wrinkle the forehead on the right side. This spontaneously resolved after a few hours.

5. Syndromes with head and neck manifestations

A. Cushing syndrome
B. Down's syndrome
C. Frey's syndrome
D. Gardener's syndrome
E. Gorlin–Goltz syndrome
F. Melkersson–Rosenthal syndrome
G. Peutz–Jeghers syndrome
H. Pierre Robin syndrome
I. Sturge–Weber syndrome
J. Treacher Collins syndrome

For each of the clinical scenarios described next, choose the SINGLE most likely syndrome from the aforementioned list. Each option may be used once, more than once, or not at all.

1. Three years post orthognathic surgery, a patient develops sweating, warmth, and flushing in the pre-auricular area worse during mealtimes.

2. A patient presents with an asymptomatic bony lump on the right angle of the mandible. Their medical history revealed regular colonoscopy for benign intestinal tumours. Radiological investigations of the head reviewed multiple osteomas, odontomas, and impacted supernumerary teeth.

3. A patient presents a right-sided mandibular jaw swelling first noticed about 6 months ago. This prompted radiological investigations of the head and jaws revealing calcification of the falx cerebri and multiple multilocular radiolucencies, respectively.

4. At a routine dental appointment, a young child is noticed to have perioral pigmentation. His oral health is otherwise good. He has a history of recurrent abdominal pain due to multiple gastrointestinal polyps.

5. While on an elective visit, you observed a young child with a markedly retruded mandible, hypoplastic zygoma, downslanting palpebral fissures, and a deformed ear.

6.   **Mechanisms of action of medications used for managing medical emergencies in dentistry**

A. Activates guanylate cyclase resulting in calcium ion release and relaxation of smooth muscle cell

B. Antiplatelet via inhibiting ADP-induced binding of fibrinogen to platelets

C. Antiplatelet via irreversible inactivation of the cyclooxygenase (COX) enzyme

D. Down-regulates the release of histamine, tryptase, and other inflammatory mediators from mast cells and basophils

E. Increases the activity of neurotransmitter gamma-aminobutyric acid (GABA)

F. Induces the formation of Phosphorylase A, which is responsible for the release of glucose-1-phosphate from glycogen polymer

G. Inhibits Na^+/K^+-ATPase causing increased intracellular calcium and cardiac contractility

H. Inhibits sustained repetitive firing by blocking use-dependent sodium channels

I. Stimulates α and β_1 adrenergic receptors

J. Stimulates β_2 adrenergic receptors

For each of the medical emergency medications next, select the SINGLE most likely mechanism of action from the previous list. Each option may be used once, more than once, or not at all.

1. Adrenaline

2. Salbutamol

3. Glyceryl trinitrate

4. Aspirin

5. Midazolam

7. **Route of administration of medical emergency medications in general dental practice**

A. Buccal
B. Inhalation
C. Intralesional
D. Intramuscular
E. Intrathecal
F. Intravascular
G. Intravenous
H. Nasal
I. Subcutaneous
J. Sublingual

For each of the medical emergency medications used in general dental practice listed next, choose the SINGLE most likely route of administration from the list. Each option may be used once, more than once, or not at all.

1. Midazolam
2. Glucose gel
3. Glucagon
4. Oxygen
5. Salbutamol

8. **Dental aspects of systemic disease**

   A. Addison's disease
   B. Hypercholesterolaemia
   C. Hypoparathyroidism
   D. Hypothyroidism
   E. Pernicious anaemia
   F. Peutz–Jeghers syndrome
   G. Plummer–Vinson/Patterson Kelly syndrome
   H. Primary hyperparathyroidism
   I. Secondary hyperparathyroidism
   J. Systemic amyloidosis

   For each of the clinical scenarios described next, select the SINGLE most likely systemic disease from the previous list. Each option may be used once, more than once, or not at all.

   1. A patient presents bilateral oral mucosa hyperpigmentation. Further investigation on referral to hospital revealed a significantly raised adrenocorticotropic hormone (ACTH) levels among other findings.

   2. A patient receives a 3-monthly intramuscular injection to manage their oral dysesthesia and episodes of numbness/tingling sensations in the hands and feet.

   3. A patient presents soreness in her mouth described as burning alongside difficulty swallowing. On examination they have bilateral angular stomatitis, a depapillated red tongue, and indented spoon-shaped fingernails.

   4. A patient with end-stage kidney disease and on dialysis has grossly enlarged bony swellings in both jaws. Imaging revealed multilocular lesions affecting the jaws and cervical spine.

   5. A patient develops numbness and tingling sensations in the perioral areas after a total thyroidectomy.

9. **Tongue changes associated with systemic disease**

   A. Black hairy tongue
   B. Blue tongue
   C. Congested tongue
   D. Enlarged tongue
   E. Fissure red lobulated tongue
   F. Geographic tongue
   G. Hyperpigmented tongue
   H. Smooth beefy red tongue
   I. Sore tongue
   J. Strawberry tongue

   For each of the clinical scenarios next, choose the SINGLE most likely associated tongue change from this list. Each option may be used once, more than once, or not at all.

   1. A patient complains of headaches with visual disturbances and enlarged lower jaw with increasing spacing between their teeth.

   2. A patient had a tongue biopsy reported as staining with Congo red and exhibiting an apple-green birefringence when viewed under polarized light.

   3. A vegetarian patient with fatigue, malaise, and headaches has been diagnosed with macrocytic anaemia.

   4. An immunocompromised patient with widespread oral thrush.

   5. A child with cretinism.

10. Head and neck oncology

A. Adenoid cystic carcinoma
B. Basal cell carcinoma
C. Giant cell tumour
D. Multiple myeloma
E. Nasopharyngeal carcinoma
F. Neurofibromatosis
G. Osteomas
H. Pleomorphic adenoma
I. Squamous cell carcinoma
J. Squamous cell papilloma

For each of the clinical scenarios next, choose the SINGLE most likely associated head and neck tumour from this list. Each option may be used once, more than once, or not at all.

1. A patient notices a slow growing, asymptomatic lump at the angle of the jaw. This is been present for more than 18 months.

2. A patient who is a farmer has slow growing persistent, painless, and non-healing ulcer on the side of the nose.

3. A patient with widespread multiple papilloma-like lesions, also has café-au-lait spots on the torso which have been present since birth.

4. A patient with longstanding pea sized bony lumps on both sides of the lingual aspect of the anterior mandible finds it difficult to wear their lower denture.

5. A patient presents with spontaneous gingival bleeding. They have a recent history of increasing thirst, bone pain, and severe malaise. Routine blood investigation shows raised serum calcium and normal blood sugar.

11. Oral side effect of systemic medications

A. Angular stomatitis
B. Erythema multiforme
C. Gingival enlargement
D. Lichenoid reaction
E. Pseudomembranous candidiasis
F. Recurrent oral ulceration
G. Sialorrhoea
H. Taste disturbances
I. Tooth discolouration
J. Xerostomia

For each of the medications next, select the SINGLE most likely oral side effect associated with their use from the previous list. Each option may be used once, more than once, or not at all.

1. Beclomethasone inhaler

2. Nifedipine

3. Bendroflumethiazide

4. Amitriptyline

5. Tetracycline

12. Management of medical problems in a dental setting

A. Consult a dermatologist
B. Discharge the patient
C. Prescribe amoxicillin
D. Prescribe metronidazole
E. Prescribe NSAIDs
F. Prescribe paracetamol
G. Refer to emergency department
H. Refer to general practitioner for medication review
I. Refer to infectious disease unit
J. Refer to ophthalmologist urgently

For each of the clinical scenario next, select the SINGLE most likely management plan best suited for each patient from the list. Each option may be used once, more than once, or not at all.

1. A patient presents recurrent oral ulceration and is on aspirin 75 mg, ramipril 2.5 mg, simvastatin 40 mg, ferrous sulphate 200 mg, and nicorandil 10 mg.

2. You suspect a patient with an acutely red eye and a cluster of vesicles restricted to his right forehead area only has herpes zoster.

3. After an anaphylactic reaction which was successfully treated in the dental practice.

4. A patient with acute dentoalveolar abscess and systemic symptoms requires urgent antibiotic treatment. He is on 5 mg warfarin daily and has no known drug allergies.

5. A patient with a history of peptic ulceration requires over-the-counter medication for pain relief for severe toothache.

13. Special investigations

A. Activated partial thromboplastin time (APTT)
B. Biopsy
C. Blood glucose diary
D. Bone profile
E. Cone beam computed tomography
F. Haemoglobin electrophoresis
G. Hb_{A1c}
H. International normalized ratio (INR)
I. Mouth swabs
J. Sickle solubility test

For each of the clinical scenario next, select the SINGLE most likely special investigation required to arrive at a diagnosis from this list. Each option may be used once, more than once, or not at all.

1. A young boy has a history of frequent epistaxis, lacerations, lip ecchymosis, and swollen painful joints. Their platelet count and bleeding time are both normal.

2. A Gambian child who has regular transfusions requires surgical extraction of a supernumerary tooth under general anaesthesia.

3. A type II diabetic has multiple periodontal abscesses despite regular dental check-ups. You are concerned about their blood glucose control.

4. A general dental practitioner (GDP) refers a patient with a persistent asymptomatic white patch at the angle of the mouth.

5. Dental imaging of a 55-year-old man's mandible reveals widespread cotton wool appearance.

14. Clinical equipment

A. Blood glucometer
B. Cotton wool
C. Nasopharyngeal airway
D. Oro-pharyngeal airway
E. Oxygen face (non-rebreathable) mask
F. Peak expiratory flow meter
G. Pocket mask with oxygen port
H. Pulse oximeter
I. Spacer device
J. Tuning fork

For each of the clinical task next, choose the SINGLE most likely option from the aforementioned list. Each option may be used once, more than once, or not at all.

1. Assess light touch in a patient with left forehead herpes zoster
2. The correct size is selected by measuring from the corner of the mouth to the angle of the mandible
3. An airway adjunct during an asthmatic attack in a child
4. Maintain airway patency in an unconscious patient
5. Assess oxygen saturation during intravenous sedation

15. Endocrine disorders

A. Acromegaly

B. Addison's disease

C. Cushing's disease

D. Diabetes insipidus

E. Diabetes mellitus

F. Hyperaldosteronism

G. Hyperparathyroidism

H. Hyperthyroidism

I. Hypothyroidism

J. Phaeochromocytoma

For each of the clinical findings next, select the SINGLE most likely associated endocrine disorder from this list. Each option may be used once, more than once, or not at all.

1. Macroglossia, malocclusion, arthralgia, headaches, and impaired glucose tolerance

2. Macroglossia, non-pitting oedema, depression, and puffy eyelids

3. Polyuria, polydipsia, thirst, irritability, and hypernatraemia

4. Polyuria, polydipsia, thirst, cramps, paraesthesia, and hypokalaemia

5. Polyuria, thirst, abdominal pain, depression, and duodenal ulcers

16. Investigating head and neck swellings

A. Contrast imaging studies
B. Excisional biopsy
C. Fine needle aspiration cytology
D. Incisional biopsy
E. Magnetic resonance imaging
F. Positron emission tomography—computed tomography
G. QuantiFERON test
H. Thyroid function test
I. Transillumination test
J. Ultrasound and core biopsy

For each of the clinical scenarios next, select the SINGLE most likely special investigation required to establish a definitive diagnosis from this list. Each option may be used once, more than once, or not at all.

1. A patient has a painless, slow growing swelling at the angle of the jaw just behind and below the lower aspect of the ear.

2. An infant is born with a large soft, lobulated, and fluctuant lump on the posterior aspect of the neck.

3. A patient with a longstanding cough and a previous episode of aspiration pneumonia is found to regurgitate undigested food.

4. A patient who has a large haemangiomatous lesion affecting the tongue is found to have an extensive network of feeding vessels in the floor of the mouth, soft palate, and oropharynx.

5. A patient complaining of weight loss, increasingly anxiety, and inability to sleep is found to have a lump in the midline of the neck.

17. Medications

A. Azathioprine
B. Ciclosporin
C. Corticosteroids
D. Cyclophosphamide
E. Diclofenac
F. Ibuprofen
G. Methotrexate
H. Mycophenolate mofetil
I. Paracetamol
J. Tacrolimus

For each of the clinical scenarios that follow, select the SINGLE most likely medication referred to from this list. Each option may be used once, more than once, or not at all.

1. A patient with chronic obstructive pulmonary disease (COPD) suffers from bone pain. A DEXA scan indicates severe osteopenia.

2. A patient with a chronic autoimmune disease develops renal failure. Oral examination revealed enlarged firm gingiva.

3. A patient with chronic rhinosinusitis and asthma requires pain relief following a left knee injury.

4. A patient with chronic immune related disease has uveitis, oral ulceration, and skin lesions. After starting medication, they develop a low white cell count.

5. A patient on medication for the management of rheumatoid arthritis is also taking folic acid supplements.

18. Mental health

A. Anorexia nervosa
B. Bulimia nervosa
C. Depression
D. Generalized anxiety disorder
E. Hypochondriasis
F. Mania
G. Obsessive compulsive disorder
H. Phobia
I. Schizophrenia
J. Temporomandibular joint dysfunction

For each of the clinical scenarios listed next, select the SINGLE most likely psychiatric disorder from the list. Each option may be used once, more than once, or not at all.

1. A patient with poor oral hygiene and badly broken-down teeth is convinced that only prophets are ordained to have similar teeth. They have a history of persistent marijuana abuse.

2. A patient with mouth ulcers seeks repeated advice about probable oral cancer. Repeated reassurances from the dental specialist appear to have no effect on their health-related anxiety.

3. A patient requires benzodiazepine premedication, prior to routine dental care.

4. An anxious patient complains of severe and persistent burning sensations in their mouth. This doesn't impact on their sleep. Repeated oral examination and special investigations are unremarkable.

5. A patient perceives that they have halitosis. To combat this, they use a mouthwash more than 30 times a day.

19. Pathogens associated with orofacial lesions

A. *Actinomyces Israeli*
B. Coxsackie virus
C. Epstein –Barr virus
D. Herpes simplex virus
E. Herpes zoster virus
F. Paramyxovirus
G. *Staphylococcus aureus*
H. *Streptococcus viridians*
I. *Toxoplasmosis gondii*
J. *Treponema palladium*

For each of the clinical scenarios to follow, choose the SINGLE most likely causative/ associated pathogen from this list. Each option may be used once, more than once, or not at all.

1. A complete denture wearer with bilateral angular stomatitis.

2. A patient with a right submandibular swelling that has multiple sinuses producing a granular and purulent discharge.

3. A young boy presents with fever, malaise, and tender enlarged parotids.

4. An immunocompromised patient with a bilateral linear white lesion along the lateral border of the tongue which doesn't rub off.

5. A young woman presents with a painless rolled ulcer on their lower lip. This is followed a month later by fever and a widespread morbilliform rash.

20. Morbidity in the elderly patient

A. Alzheimer's disease
B. Benign prostatic hypertrophy
C. Chronic kidney disease
D. Gout arthritis
E. Huntington's disease
F. Multi-infarct dementia
G. Osteoarthritis
H. Parkinson's disease
I. Rheumatoid arthritis
J. Vascular dementia

For each of the clinical scenarios listed next, choose the SINGLE most likely corresponding item from this list. Each option may be used once, more than once, or not at all.

1. A patient has hands tremors worse at rest but disappear on voluntary movement.

2. A patient experiences incomplete emptying and terminal dribbling after using the bathroom. He has a previous history of urgent catheter insertion to help relieve his inability to pass urine.

3. A patient with a history of several transient ischaemic attacks finds it difficult to maintain her concentration. Lately, they have problems recalling recent events.

4. An arthritic patient with generalized pain and difficulty holding knife and fork to eat. Hand imaging revealed subluxation of the metacarpophalangeal joint and ulnar deviation.

5. An arthritic patient notices increasingly painful nodules at the terminal interphalangeal joint of their fingers. Imaging reveals interphalangeal erosion and osteophyte formation.

EMQ ANSWERS, RATIONALE, AND FURTHER READING

Introduction

Answers, feedback, and explanations demonstrating why the correct answer is most plausible and other options are incorrect is provided in this chapter. Sign-posting to other sources of further information such as the *Oxford Handbook of Clinical Medicine*, websites, and journal articles is also provided in this chapter.

Answers

1. Recognition of a patient's medication use

1. J Onset of diabetes at a young age suggests this patient's diabetes mellitus is type 1, i.e. insulin dependent (IDDM). Type 1 diabetes is an autoimmune condition which results in the destruction of B-islet cells responsible for insulin production. To compensate for the absence of endogenous insulin, these patients require regular subcutaneous injection of insulin which is usually self-administered. Preferred sites for injection include the abdomen, anterolateral aspect of the thigh, etc.

Further reading

Scully C. Chapter 6: Endocrinology. In: Scully C (ed.). *Scully's Medical Problems in Dentistry*, 7th Edition. Edinburgh, UK: Churchill Livingston/Elsevier, 2014.

2. E Multiple sclerosis is a chronic relapsing autoinflammatory T-cell-mediated immune disease which affects young adults. It causes multiple discrete plaques of demyelination that ultimately heal by scarring. This affects the white matter of the central nervous system and can occur at different sites. The majority of patients with multiple sclerosis have the relapsing-remitting disease type. The acute phase of the disease is typically managed with immunosuppressant medication, i.e. high-dose corticosteroids (intravenous methylprednisolone) to manage symptoms and ultimately shorten disease relapses.

Further reading

Wilkinson IB, Raine T, Wiles K, Goodhart A, Hall C, O'Neill H. Chapter 10: Neurology. In: Wilkinson IB, *et al.* (eds). *Oxford Handbook of Clinical Medicine*, 10th Edition. Oxford, UK: Oxford University Press, 2019.

3. F Patients with a history of bone metastases following breast cancer will be managed with intravenous bisphosphonates (antiresorptive medications) to improve their quality of life. Current guidelines aimed at preventing medication induced osteoradionecrosis of the jaw (MRONJ) recommend prior consultation with the dental profession and the use of appropriate preventative dental measures before commencing antiresorptive therapy. This is to ensure teeth with poor prognosis are extracted and their sockets are healed prior to commencing therapy. Furthermore, the preventative measures aim to maintain the teeth and supporting structures, thereby minimizing the need for surgical intervention.

Further reading

American Association of Oral and Maxillofacial Surgeons. *Medication-Related Osteonecrosis of the Jaw— 2014 Update*. 2014. Available at: https://www.aaoms.org/images/uploads/pdfs/mronj_position_paper. pdf

4. I Applying Surgicel, suturing the tooth socket to control bleeding after an emergency extraction, and a history of atrial fibrillation suggest this patient is on an anticoagulant drug. Rivaroxaban is the only oral anticoagulant in the list of options.

Further reading

National Institute for Health and Care Excellence (NICE). Atrial fibrillation: management. Clinical guideline [CG180]. 2014. Available at: https://www.nice.org.uk/guidance/cg180/chapter/Introduction

5. C A history of bleeding on brushing only in a 40-year-old is suggestive of chronic periodontitis. This can be managed with a scale and polish and appropriate oral hygiene measures, i.e. the use of mouthwashes, etc. The most likely mouthwash to cause yellowish discolouration of the patient's teeth is chlorhexidine, i.e. Corsodyl mouthwash. The other mouthwashes in the options are Difflam, benzydamine, used as a topical analgesic and betamethasone, used as a topical anti-inflammatory.

Further reading

Oral B. Chlorhexidine mouthwash: pros and cons. (n.d.) Available at: https://oralb.com/en-us/oral-health/solutions/mouthwash/chlorhexidine-mouthwash-pros-and-cons

2. Recognition of a patient's morbidities

1. I Stevens–Johnson syndrome is a severe form of erythema multiforme. It can be triggered by a hypersensitive reaction to drugs (sulphonamides, non-steroidal anti-inflammatory drugs (NSAIDs), carbamazepine, and phenytoin) or infections (herpes simplex virus, mycoplasma). Patients usually present with prodromal symptoms like fever, malaise arthralgia, myalgia, and mucosal involvement (genital, mouth, and eye ulcers). Target lesions, i.e. an area of erythema with a central blister, are seen on the palm/soles, limbs, and other parts of the skin. The disease is self-limiting so removing any precipitant and supportive care may help.

Further reading

Wilkinson IB, Raine T, Wiles K, Goodhart A, Hall C, O'Neill H. Chapter 12: Rheumatology. In: Wilkinson IB, *et al.* (eds). *Oxford Handbook of Clinical Medicine*, 10th Edition. Oxford, UK: Oxford University Press, 2019.

2. F Crohn's and ulcerative colitis are both classified as inflammatory bowel disease. Ulcerative colitis is characterized by diffuse inflammation affecting the mucosa of the colon only, whereas Crohn's disease involves patchy transmural ulceration which can affect any part of the gastrointestinal tract. Ninety per cent of patients with ulcerative colitis are likely to report bloody diarrhoea; other symptoms include abdominal pain and urgency of defecation. In Crohn's disease, patients experience chronic diarrhoea, abdominal pain, and weight loss. Blood investigations in both groups of patients may reveal microcytosis suggestive of iron deficiency anaemia or anaemia of chronic disease and thrombocytosis indicative of inflammation. Faecal calprotectin is released into the colon in excess in the presence of inflammation. National Institute for Health and Care Excellence (NICE) stipulates that the faecal calprotectin test may be helpful in distinguishing inflammatory bowel disease from other non-inflammatory bowel disease like irritable bowel syndrome, especially where lower gastrointestinal symptoms are of recent onset.

Further reading

Mozdiak E, O'Malley J, Arasaradnam R. Inflammatory bowel disease. *BMJ*, 2015;351:h4416.

3. D The patient's signs and symptoms are suggestive of liver disease. An unremarkable social history, i.e. no history of drinking alcohol or smoking, no intravenous drug abuse, married, heterosexual sexual orientation, and no recent travel abroad excludes alcoholic liver disease, hepatitis A, B, and C. Obesity, type II diabetes, and a significantly raised aspartate aminotransferase (AST) make fatty liver disease the single most likely answer.

Further reading

Wilkinson IB, Raine T, Wiles K, Goodhart A, Hall C, O'Neill H. Chapter 6: Gastroenterology. In: Wilkinson IB, *et al.* (eds). *Oxford Handbook of Clinical Medicine*, 10th Edition. Oxford, UK: Oxford University Press, 2019.

4. A Lethargy and low mood suggest this patient may be hypothyroid or has Addison's disease or is becoming addisonian. However, the patient's unexplained abdominal pain, vomiting, low glucose levels, and hyperkalaemia make Addison's disease the single most correct option.

Further reading

Wilkinson IB, Raine T, Wiles K, Goodhart A, Hall C, O'Neill H. Chapter 5: Endocrinology. In: Wilkinson IB, *et al.* (eds). *Oxford Handbook of Clinical Medicine*, 10th Edition. Oxford, UK: Oxford University Press, 2019.

5. H Multiple sclerosis patients can present trigeminal neuralgia features, as is the case with this patient's facial pain. The sudden onset of unilateral eye pain, i.e. optic neuritis, blurred vision, and bilateral presentation on both left and right sides of the face, makes multiple sclerosis the most correct option.

Further reading

Wilkinson IB, Raine T, Wiles K, Goodhart A, Hall C, O'Neill H. Chapter 10: Neurology. In: Wilkinson IB, *et al.* (eds). *Oxford Handbook of Clinical Medicine*, 10th Edition. Oxford, UK: Oxford University Press, 2019.

3. Therapeutics

1. I Asthmatics carry an increased risk of developing aspirin sensitivity compared to the general population. This can manifest as urticaria, angioedema, or rhinitis, and exacerbation of a pre-existing asthma following aspirin ingestion. NSAIDs which inhibit cyclooxygenase display similar characteristics because of a high incidence of cross-sensitivity. Therefore, paracetamol will be the analgesic of choice because it is well tolerated by the majority of patients with asthma and is seldom associated with cross-sensitivity.

Further reading

Jenkins C. Recommending analgesics for people with asthma. *Am J Ther*, 2000;7(2):55–61.

2. A The elevated temperature and evidence of local and systemic spread of the dentoalveolar abscess in this patient warrants the use of an appropriate systemic antimicrobial as adjuncts to the definitive management which could be drainage of the associated abscess, removal of the infected pulp content, or extraction of the tooth. Three choices of antibiotics are available: first choice is penicillin, e.g. amoxicillin, second choice is metronidazole, and the third choice is a macrolide, clarithromycin, azithromycin, or erythromycin. Metronidazole is contraindicated because the patient is an alcoholic; taking alcohol with metronidazole can precipitate a disulfiram-like reaction. The macrolides are reserved for patients who are allergic to penicillin. Therefore, amoxicillin is the antibiotic of choice. *Note*: prescribing a cephalosporin (e.g. cefalexin) offers no advantage over penicillin and inappropriate use can contribute to the development of resistance to the drug.

This patient can be safely prescribed amoxicillin 500 mg three times daily for up to 5 days.

Further reading

Palmer NOA, et al. *Antimicrobial Prescribing for General Dental Practitioners*, 2nd Edition. London, UK: Faculty of General Dental Practitioners (FGDP), 2014.

3. H The presence of an asymptomatic white patch at the corners of the mouth which cannot be rubbed off in a smoker is suggestive of chronic hyperplastic candidiasis. This can be managed by removing the underlying cause, i.e. smoking cessation and treatment with an appropriate antifungal medication. Because this patient is on warfarin, azole antifungals are contraindicated. A suitable alternative is the use of polyene antifungals (Nystatin oral suspensions).

This patient can be safely prescribed Nystatin oral suspension 100,000 units/ml four times daily after food for 7 days, or continued for 2 days after the lesion has healed.

Further reading

Gov.uk. *Drug Safety Update: Topical Miconazole, Including Oral Gel: Reminder of Potential for Serious Interactions with Warfarin.* London, UK: Medicine and Healthcare Products Regulatory Agency (MHRA), 15 June 2016. Available at: https://www.gov.uk/drug-safety-update/topical-miconazole-including-oral-gel-reminder-of-potential-for-serious-interactions-with-warfarin

4. E The first line of treatment for patients who are allergic to penicillin is metronidazole. It can also be used as first line treatment in patients who have had a recent course of penicillin for another infection or if a predominantly anaerobic infection is suspected or microbiologically proven.

This patient can be safely prescribed metronidazole 400 mg three times daily for up to 5 days; review after 2–3 days and discontinue if resolved.

Further reading

Palmer NOA, *et al. Antimicrobial Prescribing for General Dental Practitioners*, 2nd Edition. London, UK: Faculty of General Dental Practitioners (FGDP), 2014.

5. J Ramipril is an angiotensin-converting enzyme (ACE) inhibitor indicated for management of hypertension, symptomatic heart failure, etc. A possible oral side effect can be the development of ulcers in the mouth. If ramipril is implicated as the cause of the patient's oral ulceration, it will be prudent to refer to the general medical practitioner or cardiologist for an alternative antihypertensive. Nifedipine, a calcium channel blocker, is a suitable alternative.

Further reading

Wakefield YS, Theaker ED, Pemberton MN. Angiotensin converting enzyme inhibitors and delayed onset, recurrent angioedema of the head and neck. *Br Dent J*, 2008;205:553–6.

4. Cranial nerve abnormalities

1. E This patient appears to be experiencing an unpleasant condition called trigeminal neuralgia. Patients suffer spasms of violent pain in the area of distribution of one of the divisions of cranial nerve V (trigeminal nerve) which is set-off by touching a trigger area. The temporary pain relief from the administration of a right infraorbital nerve block suggests the right maxillary division of the trigeminal nerve is the most likely to be affected.

Further reading

Scully C. Chapter 13: Neurology. In: Scully C (ed.). *Scully's Medical Problems in Dentistry*, 7th Edition. Edinburgh, UK: Churchill Livingston/Elsevier, 2014.

2. E This patient appears to be experiencing shingles (*herpes zoster*) involving the ophthalmic division of cranial nerve V (trigeminal nerve). Herpes zoster is caused by reactivation of the virus, which lies in the sensory nerve ganglia following a previous infection of chicken pox. Because this can result in permanent impairment of vision, it is treated as an ophthalmological emergency.

Further reading

Wilkinson IB, Raine T, Wiles K, Goodhart A, Hall C, O'Neill H. Chapter 9: Infectious diseases. In: Wilkinson IB, *et al.* (eds). *Oxford Handbook of Clinical Medicine*, 10th Edition. Oxford, UK: Oxford University Press, 2019.

3. F This patient's clinical features are suggestive of herpes zoster infection involving the geniculate ganglion of cranial nerve VII (facial nerve). This nerve supplies special taste sensations to the anterior two-thirds of the tongue via the chorda tympani nerve and to the stapedius muscle via nerve to stapedius. A defect of this nerve, evident in Ramsey–Hunt syndrome, can give rise to the patient's symptoms.

Further reading

Wilkinson IB, Raine T, Wiles K, Goodhart A, Hall C, O'Neill H. Chapter 9: Infectious diseases. In: Wilkinson IB, *et al.* (eds). *Oxford Handbook of Clinical Medicine*, 10th Edition. Oxford, UK: Oxford University Press, 2019.

4. E The axons of the motor nucleus run in the motor root of the mandibular division of cranial nerve V through which they are distributed to the muscles of mastication. Damage to the motor nucleus (trigeminal motor neuropathy) will cause weakness or paralysis of the muscles of mastication resulting in deviation to the side of the lesion on mouth opening. This is easier to detect when the patient is asked to open their jaw against resistance.

Further reading

Scully C. Chapter 13: Neurology. In: Scully C (ed.). *Scully's Medical Problems in Dentistry*, 7th Edition. Edinburgh, UK: Churchill Livingston/Elsevier, 2014.

5. F The temporary facial paralysis following administration of an inferior dental nerve block is as a result of accidental deposition of local anaesthetic solution into the parotid gland through which the facial nerve transverses. The facial nerve divides the superficial from the deep lobe of the parotid gland.

Further reading

Johnson DR, Moore WJ. *Anatomy for Dental Students*, 3rd Edition, p. 259. Oxford, UK: Oxford University Press, 1996.

5. Syndromes with head and neck manifestations

1. C The patient's clinical features are suggestive of Frey's syndrome. This can arise following a parotidectomy or trauma to the parotid area, which results in joining of damaged post-ganglionic parasympathetic nerve fibre with sympathetic nerve endings. The resultant effect is sweating and flushing of the pre-auricular skin in response to stimulation of salivation, i.e. in anticipation of food, at mealtimes, or chewing.

Further reading

Scully C. Chapter 14: Otorhinolaryngology/maxillofacial disorders. In: Scully C (ed.). *Scully's Medical Problems in Dentistry*, 7th Edition. Edinburgh, UK: Churchill Livingston/Elsevier, 2014.

2. D The clinical and radiological features are suggestive of Gardener's syndrome.

Further reading

Lee BD, Lee W, Oh SH, Min SK, Kim EC. A case report of Gardner syndrome with hereditary widespread osteomatous jaw lesions. *Oral Surg Oral Med Oral Pathol Oral Radiol Endod*, 2009;107(3):e68–e72.

3. E The clinical and radiological features are suggestive of Gorlin–Goltz syndrome (NBCCS).

Further reading

Casaroto AR, *et al.* Early diagnosis of Gorlin–Goltz syndrome: case report. *Head Face Med*, 2011;7:2.

4. G The clinical and investigation findings are suggestive of Peutz–Jeghers syndrome.

Further reading

Kopacova M, Tacheci I, Rejchrt S, Bures J. Peutz–Jeghers syndrome: diagnostic and therapeutic approach. *World J Gastroenterol*, 2009;15(43):5397–408.

5. J The characteristic facial features described are those of Treacher Collins syndrome, aka mandibulofacial dysostosis.

Further reading

Woo S-B. *Oral and Maxillofacial Pathology*, 2nd Edition, p. 42. Philadelphia, PA: Elsevier, 2016.

6. Mechanisms of action of medications used for managing medical emergencies in dentistry

1. I Adrenaline works via the stimulation of α and β-1 adrenergic receptors, with moderate activity via β-2 adrenergic receptors. These produce vasoconstriction and bronchodilation, thereby reversing the vasodilation and bronchoconstriction mediated by inflammatory mediators produced during anaphylaxis.

Further reading

BNF Publications. Available at: https://www.bnf.org

2. J Salbutamol binds to β_2-receptors in the airway causing bronchodilation via relaxation of bronchial smooth muscles.

Further reading

BNF Publications. Available at: https://www.bnf.org

3. A Glyceryl trinitrate is broken down to nitric oxide (NO), which in turn activates the enzyme guanylate cyclase. The consequence of this is the release of calcium ions, which produces relaxation of the smooth muscle cells and vasodilation.

Further reading

BNF Publications. Available at: https://www.bnf.org

4. C Aspirin directly and irreversibly inhibits the activity of COX-1 and COX-2 thereby reducing the formation of prostaglandins and thromboxanes from arachidonic acid. Both of these mediators are potent aggregators.

Further reading

BNF Publications. Available at: https://www.bnf.org

5. E Midazolam is a short-acting benzodiazepine central nervous system (CNS) depressant. Its actions are mediated through the inhibitory neurotransmitter gamma-aminobutyric acid (GABA). It increases the activity of GABA, thereby producing a calming effect, relaxing skeletal muscles, and inducing sleep.

Further reading

BNF Publications. Available at: https://www.bnf.org

7. Route of administration of medical emergency medications in general dental practice

1. A Midazolam via the buccal mucosa is route of administration recommended by the Resuscitation Council UK for management of patients with prolonged convulsive seizures (5 minutes or more) or repeated seizures (three or more in an hour) in general dental practice. Other routes of administration for midazolam include intranasal, intramuscular, and intravenous. The buccal route is preferred because it is safe, effective, and can be used with ease outside hospital (general dental practice). An additional benefit is the avoidance of embarrassment and difficulty associated with administration of rectal diazepam, a commonly used treatment for managing seizures.

Further reading

Scheepers M, Comish S, Cordes L, Clough P, Scheepers B. Buccal midazolam and rectal diazepam for epilepsy. *Lancet*, 1999;353(9166):1797–8.

2. A Glucose gel or GlucoGel is proprietary product of quick-acting carbohydrate administered by mouth for management of a conscious hypoglycaemic patient with an intact gag reflex. Alternatively, approximately 10 g of fast acting glucose is available from two teaspoons of sugar, or from three sugar lumps, and also from non-diet versions of the following soft drinks: 110 ml of Lucozade® Energy Original, 100 ml of Coca-Cola®, 19 ml of Ribena® Blackcurrant can be administered.

Further reading

National Institute for Health and Care Excellence. Hypoglycaemia. Available at: https://bnf.nice.org.uk/treatment-summary/hypoglycaemia.html

3. D Glucagon, 1 mg, via the intramuscular route is recommended for management of hypoglycaemic patients who either become unconscious and/or are unable to be given fast-acting glucose via the mouth in general dental practice. Carbohydrates should be given as soon as the patient regains consciousness and able to take glucose via mouth to restore glycogen store in the liver.

Further reading

British Dental Association (BDA). Medical emergencies in the dental practice. *BDJ Team* ISSN 2054-7617 (online). Available at: https://www.nature.com/articles/bdjteam201655/figures/1

4. B Oxygen is delivered via the inhalation route at a flow rate of 10–15 litres per minute through an oxygen face mask with oxygen reservoir and tubing (also called an oxygen non-rebreathe mask in general dental practice). Indications for emergency administration of oxygen in general dental practice include syncope, acute asthmatic attack, anaphylaxis, during an epileptic fit, and cardiopulmonary resuscitation.

Further reading

Jevon P. Emergency oxygen therapy in the dental practice. *BDJ Team*, 2015;1:14045.

5. B Salbutamol is delivered via the inhalation route, initially from the patient's inhaler if they are known asthmatics and have attended with it, or via a spacer device if the patient is unable to effectively use their inhaler. Two puffs (100 μg/puff) is recommended for the former and ten activations of the salbutamol inhaler using a spacer device. A repeat dose every 10 minutes is recommended if necessary.

Further reading

British Dental Association (BDA). Medical emergencies in the dental practice. *BDJ Team* ISSN 2054-7617 (online). Available at: https://www.nature.com/articles/bdjteam201655/figures/1

8. Dental aspects of systemic disease

1. A Bilateral oral hyperpigmentation, raised adrenocorticotropic hormone (ACTH) and low cortisol levels are characteristic of Addison's disease. The raised ACTH levels, a pituitary hormone with a chemical structure similar to that of melanocyte-stimulating hormone (MSH), is responsible for the pigmentation of the skin and mucosa.

Further reading

Wilkinson IB, Raine T, Wiles K, Goodhart A, Hall C, O'Neill H. Chapter 5: Endocrinology. In: Wilkinson IB, et al. (eds). *Oxford Handbook of Clinical Medicine*, 10th Edition. Oxford, UK: Oxford University Press, 2019.

2. E The most likely systemic disease in this patient is pernicious anaemia. Pernicious anaemia is an autoimmune disease, characterized by destruction of gastric parietal cells responsible for the production of intrinsic factor. Intrinsic factor forms a complex with vitamin B_{12}, facilitating absorption at the terminal ileum. Therefore, patients with pernicious anaemia (autoimmune gastritis) are unable to absorb B_{12} and manifest low serum levels. In the United Kingdom, 3-monthly injection of 1 mg/ml cyanocobalamin (vitamin B_{12}) is the preferred method of treatment. Although treatment with oral cyanocobalamin is also available and being advocated, the efficacy and cost-effectiveness of oral treatment in wider population-based settings has yet to be established.

Further reading

Hunt A, Harrington D, Robinson S. Vitamin B_{12} deficiency. *BMJ*, 2014;349:g5226.

Neville BW, Damm DD, Allen C, Bouquot J. Chapter 17: Oral manifestations of systemic disease. In: Neville BW, Damm DD, Allen C, Bouquot J (eds). *Oral and Maxillofacial Pathology*, 2nd Edition. Philadelphia, PA: W.B. Saunders/Elsevier, 2002.

3. G Dysphagia, brittle nails, koilonychia, diffuse papillary atrophy of tongue, angular chelitis, and burning sensation of the oral mucosa in this 55-year-old female are most likely to be associated with Plummer–Vinson syndrome (Paterson–Kelly syndrome). This condition is rare but carries a substantial risk of malignant transformation in the post-cricoid region.

Further reading

Scully C. Chapter 8: Haematology. In: Scully C (ed.). *Scully's Medical Problems in Dentistry*, 7th Edition. Edinburgh, UK: Churchill Livingston/Elsevier, 2014.

4. I The kidneys play an important role in production of active vitamin D required for calcium absorption from the gastrointestinal tract, and excretion and reabsorption of calcium and phosphate. Therefore, a patient with end-stage kidney disease on regular dialysis could develop low serum calcium. To compensate for this, they develop secondary hyperparathyroidism (increased parathormone secretion). The increased parathormone promotes osteoclastic bone resorption to prop up serum calcium levels. Long-term consequences are the development of lytic lesions (giant cell lesions) involving the jaws and cervical spine, bone rarefaction, loss of lamina dura, and pulp stones. In severe cases, as is the case in this scenario, significant expansion of the cortical plates of the jaws culminating in a reduced oral cavity can occur. Patients can also manifest the classic triad of signs and symptoms, described as stones, bones, and groans.

Further reading

Gadhia T, Adegun OK, Fortune F. Brown tumours: widespread involvement of multiple maxillofacial bones and cervical spine. *BMJ Case Rep*, 2014;2014:bcr2014207140.

5. C Iatrogenic injury of the parathyroid glands resulting in transient or permanent hypoparathyroidism is an unintended consequence of total thyroidectomy. This can be identified by measuring serum parathormone (PTH) level immediately after surgery with a view to identifying patient at risk of hypocalcaemia. Calcium and activated vitamin D are usually administered to patients with low postoperative PTH to reduce the incidence of symptomatic hypocalcaemia.

Further reading

Allweiss P, Guesto WJ, Carek PJ. Chapter 37: Endocrine disorders. In: South-Paul JE (ed.). *Current Diagnosis & Treatment in Family Medicine*, 4th Edition. New York, USA: McGraw-Hill Education/Medical, 2015.

Ritter K, Elfenbein D, Schneider DF, Chen H, Sippel RS. Hypoparathyroidism after total thyroidectomy: incidence and resolution. *J Surg Res*, 2015;197(2):348–53.

9. Tongue changes associated with systemic disease

1. D The clinical signs and symptoms in this patient are suggestive of acromegaly characterized by excess production of growth hormones after closure of the epiphyseal plates. Excessive soft tissue growth can result in an enlarged tongue (macroglossia).

Further reading

Wilkinson IB, Raine T, Wiles K, Goodhart A, Hall C, O'Neill H. Chapter 5: Endocrinology. In: Wilkinson IB, *et al.* (eds). *Oxford Handbook of Clinical Medicine*, 10th Edition. Oxford, UK: Oxford University Press, 2019.

2. D The biopsy report finding is diagnostic of amyloidosis. Macroglossia can be associated with systemic or localized amyloid deposition.

Further reading

Woo S-B. Chapter 17: Oral manifestations of systemic diseases. In: Woo S-B (ed.). *Oral and Maxillofacial Pathology*, 2nd Edition, p. 42. Philadelphia, PA: Elsevier, 2016.

3. I Fatigue, shortness of breath, and headaches are non-specific symptoms of anaemia. The patient's dietary history and macrocytic anaemia is suggestive of folate and/or vitamin B_{12} deficiency. These patients can develop a sore/burning tongue in the absence of any physical abnormality.

Further reading

Woo S-B. Chapter 17: Oral manifestations of systemic diseases. In: Woo S-B (ed.). *Oral and Maxillofacial Pathology*, 2nd Edition, p. 42. Philadelphia, PA: Elsevier, 2016.

4. I An immunocompromised patient with widespread thrush (pseudomembranous candidiasis) is most likely to present with local discomfort which can manifest as a sore tongue and altered taste sensation. Black hairy tongue is incorrect as this is not synonymous with oral hairy leukoplakia, which is associated with Epstein–Barr virus infection in immunocompromised patients.

Further reading

Akpan A, Morgan R. Oral candidiasis. *Postgrad Med J*, 2002;78(922):455–9.

5. D Cretinism refers to congenital hypothyroidism. These children can present with macroglossia (enlarged tongue).

Further reading

Gupta R, Goel K, Solanki J, Gupta S. Oral manifestations of hypothyroidism: a case report. *J Clin Diagn Res*, 2014;8(5):ZD20.

10. Head and neck oncology

1. H A slow growing, asymptomatic lump at the angle of the jaw present for more than 18 months is suggestive of a benign tumour of parotid gland. The most common benign salivary gland neoplasm is a pleomorphic adenoma. Adenoid cystic carcinoma is malignant and well known for their perineural spread and resultant facial paralysis.

Further reading

Wilkinson IB, Raine T, Wiles K, Goodhart A, Hall C, O'Neill H. Chapter 13: Surgery. In: Wilkinson IB, *et al.* (eds). Oxford Handbook of Clinical Medicine, 10th Edition. Oxford, UK: Oxford University Press, 2019.

2. B The occupation (outdoors), location of the ulcer (sun-exposed sites), and clinical manifestations make basal cell carcinoma the most likely diagnosis. Squamous cell carcinoma can also present as an ulcerated lesion, however, bleeding, induration, raised edges, metastasis to lymph nodes, and rapid lesional changes are also characteristics.

Further reading

Wilkinson IB, Raine T, Wiles K, Goodhart A, Hall C, O'Neill H. Chapter 13: Surgery. In: Wilkinson IB, *et al.* (eds). *Oxford Handbook of Clinical Medicine*, 10th Edition. Oxford, UK: Oxford University Press, 2019.

3. F These features are characteristic of neurofibromatosis specifically type 1, aka Von Recklinghausen's disease.

Further reading

Wilkinson IB, Raine T, Wiles K, Goodhart A, Hall C, O'Neill H. Chapter 10: Neurology. In: Wilkinson IB, *et al.* (eds). *Oxford Handbook of Clinical Medicine*, 10th Edition. Oxford, UK: Oxford University Press, 2019.

4. G The mandibular bony swellings on the lingual aspect of both mandibles are bony exostosis/mandibular tori/osteomas. They can impede denture wearing.

Further reading

Scully C. Chapter 37: Eponymous and acronymous diseases.. In: Scully C (ed.). *Scully's Medical Problems in Dentistry*, 7th Edition. Edinburgh, UK: Churchill Livingston/Elsevier, 2014.

5. D The clinical features and blood investigation findings are characteristic of multiple myeloma.

Further reading

Wilkinson IB, Raine T, Wiles K, Goodhart A, Hall C, O'Neill H. Chapter 8: Haematology. In: Wilkinson IB, *et al.* (eds). *Oxford Handbook of Clinical Medicine*, 10th Edition. Oxford, UK: Oxford University Press, 2019.

11. Oral side effects of systemic medications

1. E Beclomethasone, a potent immunosuppressant, is used as a topical anti-inflammatory and in aerosol form for prophylactic management of asthma and allergic rhinitis. Thrush (acute pseudomembranous candidiasis) at the back of roof of the mouth, throat, and uvula is a common oral side effect. To avoid this, patients are advised to rinse their mouth immediately after its use or use a spacer device to minimize deposition of the medication on the oral mucosa.

Further reading

National Health Service. Steroid inhalers. Available at: https://www.nhs.uk/Conditions/steroid-inhalers/Pages/Introduction.aspx

2. C Nifedipine is a dihydropyridine calcium channel blocker. It is an antihypertensive medication. Gingival hyperplasia/hypertrophy is a common oral side effect.

Further reading

National Institute for Health and Care Excellence. Nifedipine. Available at: https://bnf.nice.org.uk/drug/nifedipine.html#sideEffects

3. D Bendroflumethiazide is a common diuretic used for management of hypertension. Patients typically used 2.5 mg daily. Common oral side effects include lichenoid reaction and ulceration. Patients typically describe the lesion as burning on eating spicy food. It typically presents on the buccal mucosa as a fine lacy white network of striae on an erythematous background.

Further reading

National Institute for Health and Care Excellence. Bendroflumethiazide. Available at: https://bnf.nice.org.uk/drug/bendroflumethiazide.html

4. J Amitriptyline is an antidepressant medication that can be used to manage a variety of conditions including neuropathic pain, migraine prophylaxis, depressive illness, etc. Xerostomia is a common oral side effect.

Further reading

Scully C. Chapter 29: Materials and drugs. In: Scully C (ed.). *Scully's Medical Problems in Dentistry*, 7th Edition. Edinburgh, UK: Churchill Livingston/Elsevier, 2014.

5. I Tetracycline is a broad-spectrum antibiotic which exerts a bacteriostatic effect by binding reversibly to the bacterial 30S ribosomal subunit and blocking incoming aminoacyl tRNA from binding to the ribosome acceptor site. It is contraindicated in pregnant women and children up to age 8 to avoid permanent discoloration of developing teeth. The discolouration can vary from yellow or grey to brown.

Further reading

Sánchez AR, Rogers RS 3rd, Sheridan PJ. Tetracycline and other tetracycline-derivative staining of the teeth and oral cavity. *Int J Dermatol*, 2004;43(10):709–15.

12. Management of medical problems in a dental setting

1. H The patient is on the following medications: antiplatelet, antihypertensive, treatment for iron deficiency anaemia, hypercholesterolaemia. Assuming no cause for the patient's oral ulceration can be identified, the most appropriate management plan will be to recommend the GP or cardiologist carry out a medication review with a view to seeking suitable alternatives for nicorandil and ramipril. Both medications can cause oral ulceration as a side effect.

Further reading

Jinbu Y, Demitsu T. Oral ulcerations due to drug medications. *Japanese Dental Science Review*, 2014;50(2):40–6.

2. J Herpes zoster involving the ophthalmic division (V1) of the trigeminal nerve can be complicated by keratitis, corneal ulceration, iridocyclitis, glaucoma, and blindness. It is an ophthalmological emergency, therefore necessitates urgent referral to an ophthalmologist.

Further reading

Ganda K. Section XIV, Chapter 47: Human immunodeficiency virus, Herpes simplex and Zoster, Lyme Disease, MRSA infection and sexually transmitted disease. In: Ganda K (ed.). *Dentist's Guide to Medical Conditions, Medications and Complications*, 2nd Edition, New York, USA: Wiley Blackwell, 2013.

3. G The likelihood of a rebound attack after successful management and initial recovery from an anaphylactic episode necessitates urgent referral to the emergency department for further management.

Further reading

Greenwood M. Chapter 21: Medical emergencies. In: Greenwood M (ed.). *Essentials of Human Disease in Dentistry*, p. 338. Hoboken, NJ: Wiley-Blackwell, 2018.

4. C Metronidazole potentiates the action of warfarin. Systemic involvement and no known drug allergies make amoxicillin, a broad-spectrum penicillin, the most suitable antibiotic to manage the patient's infection.

Further reading

Ganda K. Section II, Chapter 6: Odontogenic infections, antibiotics and infection management protocols. In: Ganda K (ed.). *Dentist's Guide to Medical Conditions, Medications and Complications*, 2nd Edition, Section XIV. New York, USA: Wiley Blackwell, 2013.

5. F Prescribing NSAIDs for pain relief can worsen the patient's peptic ulceration. Paracetamol is best suited for this patient.

Further reading

Ganda K. Section II, Chapter 5: Pain physiology, analgesics, opioid dependency maintenance therapies, multimodal analgesia and pain management algorithms. In: Ganda K (ed.). *Dentist's Guide to Medical Conditions, Medications and Complications*, 2nd Edition, Section XIV. New York, USA: Wiley Blackwell, 2013.

13. Special investigations

1. A The patient's sex, clinical features, and preliminary investigation findings are in keeping with those of a haemophilic. An activated partial thromboplastin time (APTT) which test for abnormalities in factor I, II, VIII, IX, X, XI, and XII will facilitate arrival at a definitive diagnosis. Note that haemophilic patients will have a normal international normalized ratio (INR), bleeding and thrombin time, and platelet count and a raised APTT.

Further reading

Wilkinson IB, Raine T, Wiles K, Goodhart A, Hall C, O'Neill H. Chapter 8: Haematology. In: Wilkinson IB, *et al.* (eds). *Oxford Handbook of Clinical Medicine*, 10th Edition. Oxford, UK: Oxford University Press, 2019.

2. F Patients of West African descent (Gambia) undergoing general anaesthesia must have a sickle-cell test. Sickle-cell solubility test confirms the presence of sickling but cannot distinguish between HbSS (sickle-cell anaemia) and HbAS (sickle-cell trait). Haemoglobin electrophoresis confirms the diagnosis and distinguishes between HbSS and HbAS and Hb variant. Therefore, it is imperative this investigation is performed prior to surgery, so appropriate pre- and post-anaesthetic is planned.

Further reading

Wilkinson IB, Raine T, Wiles K, Goodhart A, Hall C, O'Neill H. Chapter 8: Haematology. In: Wilkinson IB, et al. (eds). *Oxford Handbook of Clinical Medicine*, 10th Edition. Oxford, UK: Oxford University Press, 2019.

3. G Glycated haemoglobin (HbAlc) measures the mean glucose levels over the previous 8 weeks, i.e. the half-life of red blood cells. It is well established that diabetic complications increase with rising HbAlc. Therefore, a diabetic patient who is not responding to periodontal therapy and meticulous oral hygiene may require this test to establish to establish their long-term blood glucose control. *Note:* Glycated haemoglobin is reliable only when normal haemoglobin is present in red blood cells that have normal lifespans. In conditions where red cells have a shortened lifespan or a haemoglobin disorder is present, Hb_{1Ac} is unreliable.

Further reading

Wilkinson IB, Raine T, Wiles K, Goodhart A, Hall C, O'Neill H. Chapter 5: Endocrinology. In: Wilkinson IB, et al. (eds). *Oxford Handbook of Clinical Medicine*, 10th Edition. Oxford, UK: Oxford University Press, 2019.

4. B A persistent asymptomatic white patch at the angle of the mouth must be investigated further by referring the patient to a specialist for a biopsy. This will exclude a premalignant or malignant lesion.

Further reading

Kalavrezos N, Scully C. Mouth cancer for clinicians' part 8: referral. *Dent Update*, 2016;43(2):176–85.

5. D Paget's disease typically affects older people and is rarely seen in patients younger than 40 years of age. Asymptomatic disease is often discovered in radiographs taken for unrelated reasons, as is the case with this patient. Radiological (patchy sclerotic areas described as having a cotton wool appearance) and a bone profile (markedly raised alkaline phosphatase, and normal calcium and phosphate) changes are diagnostic findings. Other clinical features include bone pain, bony deformity, and enlargement typically of the pelvis, lumber spine, skull, femur, and tibia.

Further reading

Woo S-B. Chapter 14: Bone pathology. In: Woo S-B. *Oral and Maxillofacial Pathology*, 2nd Edition. Philadelphia, PA: Elsevier, 2016.

14. Clinical equipment

1. B A cotton wool swab or cotton ball is used to assess light touch. A pin prick is used to assess for pain, while a tuning fork is used for assessing temperature sensation.

Further reading

Sanders RD. The trigeminal (V) and facial (VII) cranial nerves: head and face sensation and movement. *Psychiatry (Edgmont)*, 2010;7(1):13.

2. D An oropharyngeal airway is used to maintain the patency of airway arising from airway obstruction due to relaxed upper airway muscles or airway blockage by the tongue. The correct size of an oropharyngeal airway is selected by measuring from the corner of the patient's mouth to the angle of the mandible.

Further reading

Advanced Cardiovascular Life Support (ACLS). *Effective Use of Oropharyngeal and Nasopharyngeal Airways*. Available at: https://acls.com/free-resources/knowledge-base/respiratory-arrest-airway-management/nasopharyngeal-oropharyngeal-airways

3. I A spacer device is used as an airway adjunct for inhalation of bronchodilators (salbutamol) during an asthmatic attack. It is particularly useful for children who are unable to coordinate their breathing during a medical emergency.

Further reading

Asthma UK. *Spacers*. Available at: https://www.asthma.org.uk/advice/inhalers-medicines-treatments/inhalers-and-spacers/spacers/

4. D An oropharyngeal airway is inserted to maintain airway patency in an unconscious patient. *Note*: an oropharyngeal airway is contraindicated in conscious patients with intact gag reflex.

Further reading

Advanced Cardiovascular Life Support (ACLS). *Effective Use of Oropharyngeal and Nasopharyngeal Airways*. Available at: https://acls.com/free-resources/knowledge-base/respiratory-arrest-airway-management/nasopharyngeal-oropharyngeal-airways

5. H Pulse oximeter is a non-invasive method for monitoring patient's oxygen saturation. The oxygen saturation measurement can be used as an indication of respiratory function during intravenous sedation.

Further reading

British Dental Association (BDA). *Conscious Sedation*. Available at: http://www.baos.org.uk/resources/BDAGuidanceconscious_sedation_-_nov_11.pdf

15. Endocrine disorders

1. A Acromegaly is caused by overproduction of growth hormone after the epiphyses have fused. A pituitary adenoma is a likely cause. In the head and neck, it affects the mandible, which has growth potential. Clinical findings include mandibular enlargement, which leads to prognathism (class III malocclusion), thickening of soft tissues and hands which become large and spade-like, visual defects, and severe headaches due to local pressure from the pituitary tumour on the optic chiasma and raised intracranial pressure, respectively. Other complications include diabetes mellitus, hypertension, cardiomyopathy, sleep apnoea, osteoarthritis, etc.

Further reading

Wilkinson IB, Raine T, Wiles K, Goodhart A, Hall C, O'Neill H. Chapter 5: Endocrinology. In: Wilkinson IB, *et al.* (eds). *Oxford Handbook of Clinical Medicine*, 10th Edition. Oxford, UK: Oxford University Press, 2019.

2. I Causes of hypothyroidism include Hashimoto thyroiditis, thyroid loss from surgery, medications such as carbimazole, lithium, amiodarone, irradiation of the neck. Clinical findings include weight gain, bradycardia, dry skin, hair loss, mental dullness, irritability, myxoedema, heart failure, puffy eyelids, etc. Congenital hypothyroidism is also associated with macroglossia and learning impairment.

Further reading

Wilkinson IB, Raine T, Wiles K, Goodhart A, Hall C, O'Neill H. Chapter 5: Endocrinology. In: Wilkinson IB, *et al.* (eds). *Oxford Handbook of Clinical Medicine*, 10th Edition. Oxford, UK: Oxford University Press, 2019.

3. D Diabetes insipidus is rare and is associated with posterior pituitary hypofunction. Specifically, it is caused by lack of antidiuretic hormone (ADH), which results in an inability to concentrate urine. Remember that ADH promotes water resorption in the renal tubules. Clinical findings include polyuria, persistent thirst, and polydipsia. Blood chemistry may reveal hypernatraemia.

Further reading

Wilkinson IB, Raine T, Wiles K, Goodhart A, Hall C, O'Neill H. Chapter 5: Endocrinology. In: Wilkinson IB, *et al.* (eds). *Oxford Handbook of Clinical Medicine*, 10th Edition. Oxford, UK: Oxford University Press, 2019.

4. F Primary hyperaldosteronism (Conn syndrome) is caused by tumour or hyperplasia of the adrenal cortex. Clinical findings include hypokalaemia which can induce cramps, muscle weakness, paraesthesia, polyuria, persistent thirst, polydipsia, etc.

Further reading

Wilkinson IB, Raine T, Wiles K, Goodhart A, Hall C, O'Neill H. Chapter 5: Endocrinology. In: Wilkinson IB, *et al.* (eds). *Oxford Handbook of Clinical Medicine*, 10th Edition. Oxford, UK: Oxford University Press, 2019.

5. G Hyperparathyroidism can be primary, secondary, or tertiary. Primary: parathyroid adenoma or rarely atypical adenoma or parathyroid carcinoma; Secondary: in response to low plasma calcium caused by chronic renal failure or prolonged dialysis; Tertiary: due to prolonged secondary hyperparathyroidism. Clinical findings include hypercalcaemia, renal stones, peptic ulceration, hypertension, arrhythmias, polyuria, psychiatric disorders, e.g. depression, giant cell tumours, etc. Colloquial descriptors such as stones, bones, and abdominal groans encapsulate their clinical findings.

Further reading

Wilkinson IB, Raine T, Wiles K, Goodhart A, Hall C, O'Neill H. Chapter 5: Endocrinology. In: Wilkinson IB, *et al.* (eds). *Oxford Handbook of Clinical Medicine*, 10th Edition. Oxford, UK: Oxford University Press, 2019.

16. Investigating head and neck swellings

1. J The clinical findings are those of a salivary gland swelling/neoplasm. This would be best investigated by performing an ultrasound and core biopsy under ultrasound guidance. A core biopsy is a procedure to remove a small amount of suspicious tissue with a hollow needle for histopathological evaluation. Compared to fine needle aspiration cytology (FNAC), core biopsies allow adequate tissue sampling, better diagnostic accuracy, and are used for grading, staging, and immunohistochemical studies.

Further reading

Bradley P, Beasley N, Au-Yong I. Imaging of neck lumps. *BMJ*, 2014;349:g6136.

Ferlito A, *et al.* The art of diagnosis in head and neck tumours. *Acta Oto-Laryngologica*, 2001;121(3):324–8.

2. I Cystic hygroma is usually seen in infants and its ability to transilluminate light is diagnostic.

Further reading

Bradley P, Beasley N, Au-Yong I. Imaging of neck lumps. *BMJ*, 2014;349:g6136.

Ferlito A, *et al.* The art of diagnosis in head and neck tumours. *Acta Oto-Laryngologica*, 2001;121(3):324–8.

3. A The clinical findings are those of a pharyngeal pouch. The lesion is dynamic, i.e. change in size in different position, therefore contrast imaging techniques like barium studies or videofluoroscopy are indicated.

Further reading

Bradley P, Beasley N, Au-Yong I. Imaging of neck lumps. *BMJ*, 2014;349:g6136.

Ferlito A, *et al.* The art of diagnosis in head and neck tumours. *Acta Oto-Laryngologica*, 2001;121(3):324–8.

4. E The size and extent of the haemangiomatous lesion warrants investigation with magnetic resonance imaging to establish the true extent of the lesion and monitor for changes.

Further reading

Bradley P, Beasley N, Au-Yong I. Imaging of neck lumps. *BMJ*, 2014;349:g6136.

Ferlito A, *et al.* The art of diagnosis in head and neck tumours. *Acta Oto-Laryngologica*, 2001;121:324–8.

5. H The clinical symptoms and lump in the midline of the neck are those of a thyroid gland swelling, i.e. toxic diffuse goitre. To confirm the patient's thyroid status, a thyroid function test should be requested. The most likely outcome in this patient is a raised thyroid stimulating hormone (TSH), reduced thyroxine (T4), and tri-iodothyronine (T3) levels.

Further reading

Bradley P, Beasley N, Au-Yong I. Imaging of neck lumps. *BMJ*, 2014;349:g6136.

Ferlito A, *et al.* The art of diagnosis in head and neck tumours. *Acta Oto-Laryngologica*, 2001;121.3:324–8.

17. Medications

1. C Patient with chronic obstructive pulmonary disease can be treated with a combination of corticosteroid and long-acting B_2 agonist. The corticosteroids can be administered in the form of metered dose inhalers or dry powder inhalers. Common corticosteroids used include fluticasone propionate, budesonide, and beclomethasone dipropionate. Notable side effects of prolonged use of high dose corticosteroids are osteoporosis and severe osteopenia.

Further reading

Wilkinson IB, Raine T, Wiles K, Goodhart A, Hall C, O'Neill H. Chapter 14: Clinical chemistry. In: Wilkinson IB, *et al.* (eds). *Oxford Handbook of Clinical Medicine*, 10th Edition. Oxford, UK: Oxford University Press, 2019.

2. B Ciclosporin is an immunosuppressive medication used for management of chronic autoimmune conditions and/or acute rejection following organ and/or bone marrow transplant. Common side effects include dose-related nephrotoxicity, gingival hyperplasia, hepatotoxicity, etc.

Patients have urea and electrolytes; creatinine levels and liver function tests checked every 2 weeks for 3 months to monitor for possible side effects. Subsequently, the tests are performed monthly for 3 months.

Further reading

National Institute for Health and Care Excellence (NICE). *DMARDs: Ciclosporin.* Available at: https://cks.nice.org.uk/dmards#!scenario:5

3. I NSAIDs (ibuprofen, diclofenac) can precipitate an asthmatic attack, therefore should not be prescribed in a known asthmatic patient with a history of chronic rhinosinusitis. Paracetamol is the safer alternative.

Further reading

Levy S, Volans G. The use of analgesics in patients with asthma. *Drug Safety*, 2001;24(11): 829–41.

4. A Azathioprine is an antimetabolite immunosuppressant medication used to manage a variety of conditions, including kidney transplant rejection, rheumatoid arthritis, immune-mediated severe oral ulceration, etc. Prior to administering the medication, a pretreatment blood test to measure thiopurine methyltransferase (TPMT) levels, an enzyme required for azathioprine breakdown, is done. Patients with low TPMT levels carry an increased risk of developing serious side effects, hence an alternative immunosuppressant should be considered. To monitor for side effects while on the medication, patients require full blood count and liver function tests weekly for 6 weeks, then twice-weekly until the dose is stable for 6 weeks, and then monthly. Common side effects include reduced white blood cell, neutrophil and platelet counts, raised mean cell volume, and increased AST and ALT.

Further reading

National Institute for Health and Care Excellence (NICE). *DMARDs: Azathioprine.* Available at: https://cks.nice.org.uk/dmards#!scenario:2

5. G Methotrexate, a disease-modifying antirheumatic drug (DMARD) is usually prescribed as a *once a week* treatment. It is used to manage rheumatoid arthritis, psoriatic arthritis, and vasculitides, etc. Folic acid is routinely coprescribed with methotrexate in order to reduce the likelihood of adverse effects and toxicity.

Further reading

National Institute for Health and Care Excellence (NICE). *DMARDs: Methotrexate.* Available at: https://cks.nice.org.uk/dmards#!scenario:10

18. Mental health

1. I The patient's poor oral hygiene and badly broken-down teeth highlights a diminished level of oral healthcare most likely reflective of the reduced quality of their overall personal behaviour. This in association with the persistent delusions and interpolation in their train of thoughts, i.e. being convinced that only prophets are ordained to have similar teeth is characteristic of schizophrenia. Environmental factors such as substance misuse, in this case a history of persistent marijuana abuse, is reported to increase risk of schizophrenia. While schizophrenia is the most plausible option, it is important to exclude a substance-induced psychotic disorder by obtaining a careful clinical history which may reveal onset, persistence, and cessation of symptoms to be related to the patient's marijuana use or withdrawal.

Further reading

Semple D, Smyth R. Chapter 6: Schizophrenia and related psychoses. In: Semple D, Smyth R (eds). *Oxford Handbook of Psychiatry*, 4th Edition. Oxford, UK: Oxford University Press, 2019.

2. E The central and diagnostic clinical feature for hypochondriasis is the preoccupation with the idea of having a serious medical condition, usually one which would lead to death or serious disability. They repeatedly ruminate on this possibility and insignificant bodily abnormalities, normal variants, normal functions, minor ailments will be interpreted as signs of serious disease. The patient consequently seeks medical advice and investigation but is unable to be reassured in a sustained fashion by negative investigations. For the patient in this scenario, they are preoccupied with the idea their mouth ulcers may represent oral cancer despite repeated reassurances from the dental specialist on the back of negative investigation findings.

Further reading

Semple D, Smyth R. Chapter 19: Liaison psychiatry. In: Semple D, Smyth R (eds). *Oxford Handbook of Psychiatry*, 4th Edition. Oxford, UK: Oxford University Press, 2019.

3. H This patient is receiving benzodiazepine premedication prior to dental treatment to help relieve their anxieties or alleviate their fears of visiting the dentist. Dental phobia and anxieties can be attributed to several reasons, including fear of pain, fear of injections, embarrassment, and loss of personal space, previous bad experience of dental treatment, etc. Simple inhalation sedation delivered through a nosepiece and intravenous sedation are other methods used to sedate patients who are extremely anxious about visiting the dentist or having dental treatment.

Further reading

National Health Service (NHS). Fear of the dentist. Available at: https://www.nhs.uk/live-well/healthy-body/fear-of-the-dentist-help/

4. D Generalized anxiety disorder is characterized by excessive worry and feelings of apprehension about everyday events/problems, with symptoms of muscle and psychic tension, causing significant distress/functional impairment. Severe and persistent burning sensations in the mouth with no clinically observable oral mucosal lesion and negative investigation findings is a characteristic presentation of burning mouth syndrome (BMS). Clinical observational studies have reported a linked between BMS and generalized anxiety states.

Further reading

Abetz LM, Savage NW. Burning mouth syndrome and psychological disorders. *Aust Dent J*, 2009;54:84–93.

5. G Obsessive-compulsive disorder (OCD) is a common chronic distressing disorder which frequently first occurs before the age of 25 years. It often generates considerable anxiety and may lead to depression. Obsessions may be defined as 'recurring, persisting, and distressing thoughts, images, or impulses which the affected patient recognizes as their own but may recognize them to be unreasonable or excessive'. This patient has repeated intrusive obsessive thoughts regarding bad breath (halitosis). Obsessional thoughts typically generate distressing anxiety which may be relieved by related compulsions (which may be thought of as the 'motor' component of obsessional thoughts). In this case the patient is using mouthwashes too frequently. OCD themes are numerous but may include 'checking', 'washing', and concerns about contamination. *Note*: this patient is not attributing the halitosis to possible disease which would be characteristic of hypochondriasis, rather they are taking compulsive actions to alleviate persisting thoughts. However, like hypochondriasis, the patient has made persistent attempt to seek information and reassurance about the halitosis from healthcare practitioners.

Further reading

Semple D, Smyth R. Chapter 9: Anxiety and stress-related disorders. In: Semple D, Smyth R (eds). *Oxford Handbook of Psychiatry*, 4th Edition. Oxford, UK: Oxford University Press, 2019.

19. Pathogens associated with orofacial lesions

1. G A complete denture wearer with a reduced lower facial height can develop wrinkling and skin folds at the angle of the mouth. Because of constant bathing by saliva, these may become macerated and redden resulting in angular stomatitis. *Candida albicans* and *Staphylococcus aureus* are commonly isolated in swabs from this site.

Further reading

Federico, JR, Basehore BM, and Zito, PM. "Angular Chelitis." (2019). https://www.ncbi.nlm.nih.gov/books/NBK536929/.

2. A Cervicofacial actinomycosis caused by *Actinomyces israeli* are quite uncommon, however, they can mimic more common dentoalveolar-related infection. Establishing a diagnosis is dependent on sulphur granules detection in the sinus exudate, identification in culture, and histology.

Further reading

Oostman O, Smego RA. Cervicofacial actinomycosis: diagnosis and management. *Curr Infect Dis Rep*, 7(3):170–4.

3. F Mumps is a highly contagious viral infection caused by *Paramyxovirus*. It is common in children and causes a painful swelling of the parotid glands, at the side of the face under the ears. Other symptoms include headaches, joint pain, and a fever.

Further reading

Scully C. Chapter 21: Infections and infestations. In: Scully C (ed.). *Scully's Medical Problems in Dentistry*, 7th Edition. Edinburgh, UK: Churchill Livingston/Elsevier, 2014.

4. C A furrowed, hairy white patch which doesn't rub off on the lateral border of the tongue is characteristic of oral hairy leukoplakia. This lesion is associated with Epstein–Barr virus (EBV) and occurs commonly in immunocompromised patients.

Further reading

Scully C. Chapter 20: Immunodeficiencies. In: Scully C (ed.). *Scully's Medical Problems in Dentistry*, 7th Edition. Edinburgh, UK: Churchill Livingston/Elsevier, 2014.

5. J A painless round ulcer with a raised margin and indurated base on the lower lip of a young woman fits well with primary chancre of syphilis. The chancre can also develop on the tongue, is highly infectious, and is associated with enlarged painless regional lymph nodes. The fever and morbilliform rash a month later (maculopapular rash) are signs and symptoms of secondary syphilis. It is not uncommon for secondary syphilis to develop while the chancre may still be present. Other oral lesions in secondary syphilis include painless ulcer (mucous patches and snail track ulcers), split papules, and condylomata.

Further reading

Scully C. Chapter 32: Sexual health. In: Scully C (ed.). *Scully's Medical Problems in Dentistry*, 7th Edition. Edinburgh, UK: Churchill Livingston/Elsevier, 2014.

20. Morbidity in the elderly patient

1. H Parkinson's disease is a chronic and progressive movement disorder of the CNS, which mainly affects the motor system. The substantia nigra of the basal ganglia where dopamine, a neurotransmitter which controls movement and coordination, is produced is mainly affected. Primary symptoms include tremors, characterized by rest tremors which abolished on voluntary movement, bradykinesia, rigidity, and postural instability.

Further reading

Wilkinson IB, Raine T, Wiles K, Goodhart A, Hall C, O'Neill H. Chapter 10: Neurology. In: Wilkinson IB, *et al.* (eds). *Oxford Handbook of Clinical Medicine*, 10th Edition. Oxford, UK: Oxford University Press, 2019.

2. B Benign prostatic hyperplasia/hypertrophy (BPH) is in the top 10 of the most commonly diagnosed diseases in men over the age of 50. 50%+ of men in their 50s experience BPH symptoms, while 90% of men in their 70s and 80s experience BPH symptoms. In BPH, the prostate increases in size and compresses the urethra making it difficult to urinate. Typical signs and symptoms include waking at night to urinate, frequent urination, sudden, uncontrollable urges to urinate, straining to start urinating, weak urine flow, dribbling after urination, feeling bladder is not completely empty, pain during urination. Potential complications include urinary retention, urinary tract infections, bladder stones, blood in the urine, incontinence, and decreased kidney function.

Further reading

BPH. *Patient Education Seminar: Learn About Enlarged Prostate Solutions*. Available at: http://www.urologix.com/wp-content/uploads/2014/08/Patient-Education-Presentation.pdf

3. J The patient's several episodes of mini-strokes, accompanied by the sudden onset and stepwise deterioration of memory make vascular dementia the most likely answer. Vascular dementia is the second most common type of dementia (after Alzheimer's disease) and is responsible for a quarter of all dementias.

Further reading

Alzheimer's Society. *Vascular Dementia: What Is It, and What Causes It?* Available at: https://www.Alzheimers.org.uk/info/20007/types_of_dementia/5/vascular_dementia

4. I The patient's hand features are possible chronic complication of rheumatoid arthritis. This is caused by compression of the median nerve in the wrist. The hand image findings are also typical of patients with a history of chronic rheumatoid arthritis. Other features include joint pain and swelling, stiffness, neck pain where there is involvement of the atlanto-axial joint, tiredness, painful swelling of metacarpophalangeal joints and proximal interphalangeal joints, etc.

Further reading

National Health Service. *Complications: Rheumatoid Arthritis*. Available at: http://www.nhs.uk/Conditions/Rheumatoid-arthritis/Pages/Complications.aspx

5. G Osteoarthritis is the most likely answer. The painful hand swellings in osteoarthritis patient are called Heberden's or Bouchard's nodes. Common imaging features include loss of joint space, subchondral sclerosis and cysts, and marginal osteophytes.

Further reading

Wilkinson IB, Raine T, Wiles K, Goodhart A, Hall C, O'Neill H. Chapter 12: Rheumatology. In: Wilkinson IB, *et al.* (eds). *Oxford Handbook of Clinical Medicine*, 10th Edition. Oxford, UK: Oxford University Press, 2019.

INDEX

Notes: Page numbers in *q* refer to Question and *a* refer to Answer.